A Champio[illegible] Giving Her Baby a Gift of Love

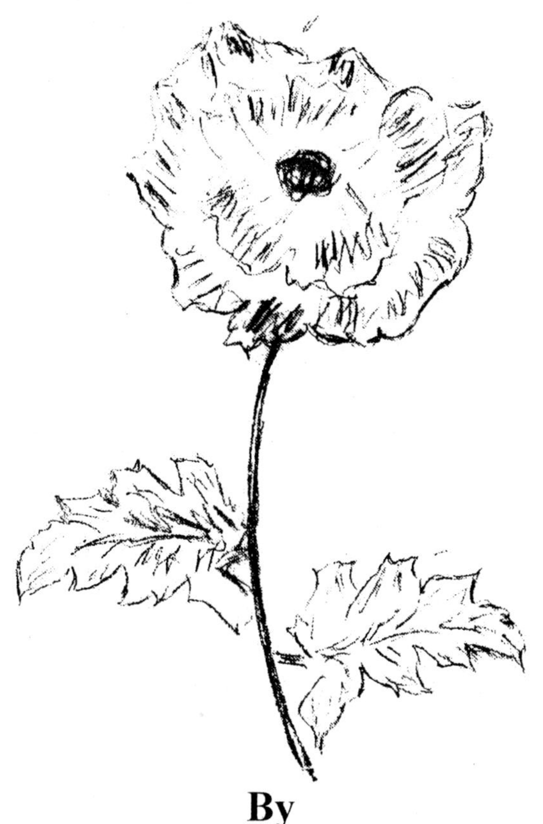

By

Gwendolyn Jackson

To Dr. Ned Robertson,
Thank you for Being such
an awesome dentist and for
your support of my book!
May God Continue to Bless
your Business!
Love
Gwendolyn
Jackson
11/28/06

ISBN: 1-4107-2371-2 (e-book)
ISBN: 1-4107-2372-0 (Paperback)

Library of Congress Control Number: 2003096221

This book is printed on acid free paper.

Printed in the United States of America
Bloomington, IN

Edited by Shirley Napier and Elizabeth McCreary

Cover Design by Dave Fair

Cover and inside photographs by Robert Hall Studios and Slimmarie Perrywatson

1stBooks - rev. 10/29/03

Acknowledgements

There are many people who contributed to this book. I am very grateful to all who had a part in helping me write this book. To my husband, George, for his prayers and patience in helping achieve this goal. To my mother, JoAnn Davis, who taught me to love and trained me in the admonition of Christ, to love God first, and live for Him always. Also, thank you for helping me with the children in order for me to work on the book and finish up last minute changes. I know that sometimes I presented challenges to situations where you did not feel up to it. Thank you for being there.

I offer special thanks to the women who took the time out of their busy schedules to share their personal testimonies and photos. I pray the best for you and your family. You have truly blessed my life. Heartfelt thanks to my photographers for taking the time out of their busy schedules to come and take various photographs and give advice without whose help this publication would not have been possible. To my spiritual mother, Shirley Napier, who took the time to help me iron out the grammar in my manuscript before submitting it-your patience to go thru it like a fine tooth comb is greatly appreciated-especially back and forth on the supplement issue. You are blessed and a precious woman of God. Hey, Dave Fair, thanks for helping at the last minute with the scanning of the photos, you are truly a blessing! To the members at Church on the Summit, thank you for your precious support. To all my friends who have supported the book, thank you.

Many thanks go to my family for their genuine support (brothers, brothers-in-law, and sisters-in-law). I send thanks to my grandmother, for showing me by example, with your life, what a real mother is suppose to be in raising her family. I love you very much. You are my inspiration in motherhood.

1st Library Books, my publisher, and Justin Axelroth, Associate Director of Author Services, thank you for your patience in working with me in all of the things it takes to make my book complete.

To my aunt Elizabeth McCreary, thank you for taking the time to proofread the manuscript and reminding me to care about important issues. You were a joyful help in turning what I wrote into English.

To my pastor, Bill and Pam McKisic, thank you for your continual prayers.

To everyone stated above, thank you for your support to make sure this book turned out well.

Ultimately, my thanks flow to my Creator, who is the source of my life.

DEDICATION

This book is dedicated to my Lord and Savior Jesus Christ. To beloved my husband for loving me and supporting me while writing this book. You are above everything my heart and soul could ever imagine being. To Jire'h who made me a mother. You are my joy. My precious daughter, Moriyah-Faith, who is a joy to look at because of your everyday smiles that sparkle through your beautiful eyes, I love you. You light up my life.

I pray that you are inspired after reading this book. And my pray is that you have a change of heart, mind, and spirit to want to do it God's way.

"You can never go back! Your baby is an infant in your life for a short time. Take advantage of the time God gives you. Children grow up fast right before your eyes!

You only get one chance to breastfeed your infant. Do not allow this precious time to pass you by; it is a gift from God!"

"I can do all things through Christ which strengtheneth me."

Philippians 4:13 KJV

Table of Contents

Author's Note:

This book has been inspired by the Holy Spirit and written as a resource for encouragement. Any information obtained here is not to be construed as medical advice. Decisions about breastfeeding should be made on an individual basis after prayer and research.

Information in this book is based on my and other mothers' experiences of breastfeeding and on the best data available during my study and research. Talk to your healthcare professional because additional information may now be available.

Foreword

Pam and I are convinced that the simple things in life are the best things in life. A beautiful sunset, the sound of gentle waves splashing on the shore, or simply a child's laughter can produce in us joy and thankfulness for the gift of life. We never cease to be amazed about the miracle of conception and birth that starts all of us on our lifelong journey. Life is so precious!

God has made such wonderful provisions for us in those first formative moments of our lives. The necessary elements of security and worth are deposited deep in our soul through the loving touch and care of our parents. This is what this book is really all about.

Gwendolyn has done a superior job in presenting the simple truth about breastfeeding. In this book, she has taken her own experience, mixed in interviews with other moms, added pros and cons, thrown in a dash of humor, and stirred it all up with the Word of God! Get ready to be both blessed and encouraged!

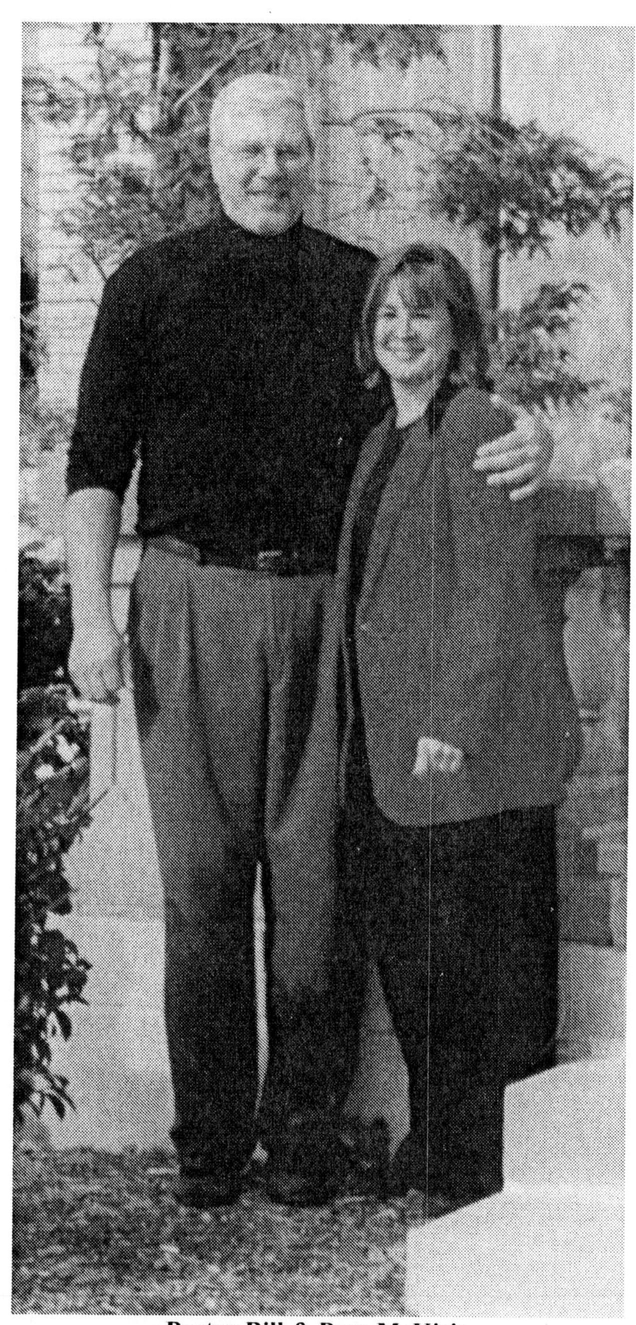

Pastor Bill & Pam McKisic
Church on the Summit, Brooklyn, Ohio

INTRODUCTION

What is a Champion Mother? **A Champion Mother is one who will go beyond the norm of society and the cares of this world to make sure that God is pleased with all they are doing where the family is concerned.**

In today's culture popular opinion tends to dictate our position in life, what to do, where to go, and what to watch and eat, to name a few. When we allow our lives to be controlled by the systematic works of society (what society considers to be the norm) we run the risk of placing material things above the needs of our children. It is our desire to encourage mothers to consider the benefits of breastfeeding and help them to make the development of their children a priority.

Your child deserves the best! As parents we must be determined to make our children's lives a priority. Parents are to take the primary responsibility in raising, training, and directing their children in the way that they should go. Breastfeeding is an excellent way to start your child off in the right direction to a healthy life.

Breastfeeding helps in the development of the child and is a treasure from God. It gives the child physical and emotional balance and strength. These are benefits that can be lost, often because we have chosen the convenience of bottle-feeding.

I believe fear takes over in many households. I mean our bills are high; and it can be tough to have to survive on only one income. There is also fear of losing your freedom (Breastfeeding does not always fit into our busy schedules.) Nursing can carry a great sacrifice of time, energy, and to our social lives. One thing is certain though; the benefits outweigh the sacrifices! A mother that is willing to sacrifice the world's way of doing things is one that will forever profit in life.

I realize that the sacrifice may fall on the husbands. Also, I realize that we are equipped to handle all that is necessary to secure families. Our wives deserve the best, and it may not come by way of acquiring all of the world's wealth or lavish homes and cars which leads to debt.

I encourage all mothers to breastfeed their children. I encourage all fathers to promote the same for their wives. Our wives' primary concern is the children and their nourishment. Meanwhile we can work for them to support their decision and desires.

God is conscious of our every need. His intent is not to take anything away from you as parents, but to allow you to see the good of your days with healthy and blessed children.

When my wife became pregnant with our son, Jire'h, it was her desire to provide the best for him. We felt that the development of our son, and of our children to come, must take priority over everything. This took sacrifice and I agreed.

When my wife and I were first married, we had an income of $80,000 between the two of us. We thought that was pretty good. But, we felt that sacrifice for the good of our child was in God's best interest and ours. So, she left her job. Knowing that it would cut our financial status in half, we decided to trust God. There were financial circumstances that challenged us. But, we believed that by making this decision we will all benefit.

My wife is a Champion Mother. Proverbs Chapter Thirty-One speaks of a woman who equipped her household with everything necessary for success. My wife reflects that. In today's society, it is refreshing to see that moral values and standards are still in existence. Thankfully, I have a wife that was willing to lose all that she worked for to nurture our son. Yes, this is rare.

She believes that God will be glorified by preparing our son and daughter with the appropriate nutrition for the development of their brain as well as their body.

As a man, a breastfeeding woman has never embarrassed me. When our son was born, he immediately took to my wife's breast as a natural. My wife nursed our son for exactly two years. The results of this are phenomenal. He is very alert, intelligent, strong and witty. I would not change the decisions we have made for the world.

When I look at all of the ills that so many children experience, I am challenged beyond one or any system that contradicts what is the best source of nourishment for a child, breast milk. I realize that there are other foods that can be given to feed a child. However, God's ways are far different than ours. He has designed it for the woman to produce nourishment to the child through the breast, not through the mass production of formulas.

I am proud of the fact that as a husband in a tainted society, God has prepared a woman to make such an awesome decision and impact on our world.

I thank God for connecting me with a Champion Mother.

George Jackson, HUSBAND

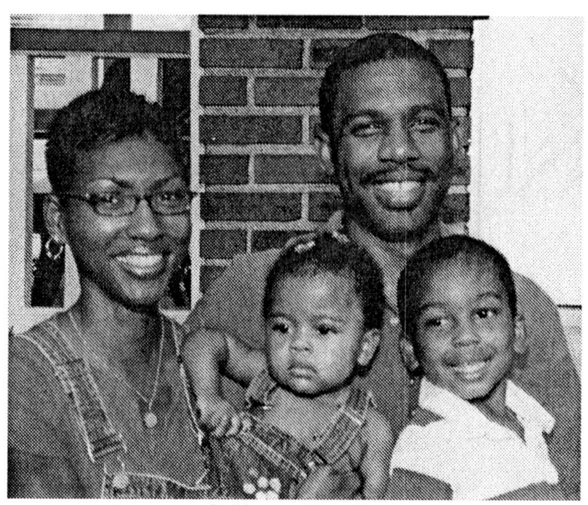

Jackson Family
George, Gwendolyn, Jiréh, Moriyah-Faith

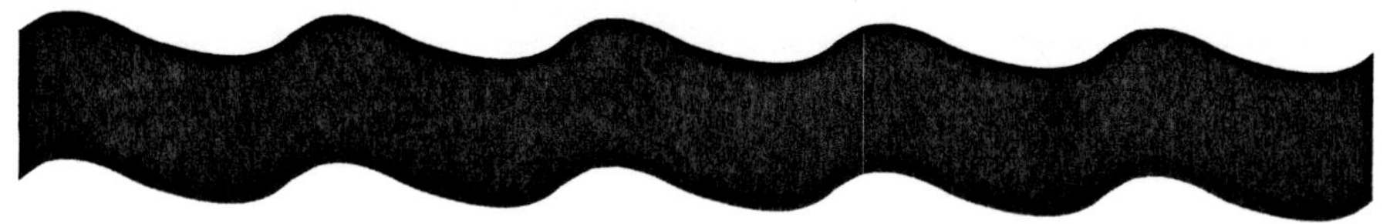

CHAPTER ONE

THE WORD OF GOD

In the Scriptures, it was the custom to breastfeed. This standard in Bible days is quite understandable. The Bible uses many scriptures in reference to nursing and weaning your baby instead of the word breastfeeding. Without the Word of God, there is no clarification and direction for a mothers' responsibility in feeding her baby. The Word of God is your stamp of approval. The words suck and suckling are used in the place of our modern word of nursing and weaned.

These are scriptures that have ministered to me when I needed strength to continue. They will also help you understand Gods perspective in this matter. There are many more scriptures that will encourage you! I pray that you will take the time to read them.

***GENESIS 21:7*.... have given children suck? ....**

***NUMBERS 11:12*... beareth the sucking child...**

***1 KINGS 3:21; 11:20*... to give my child suck, /weaned in Pharaoh's house...**

***JOB 3:12*... or why the breast that I should suck?**

***ISAIAH 60:16*... shall also suck the milk of...**

***ISAIAH 66:11, 12*... that ye may suck and be satisfied with the breast of her...**

***ISAIAH 11:8*... that ye may milk out, and be delighted...**

***ISAIAH 49:15;* ... can a woman forget her sucking child...**

***ISAIAH 28:9*... them that are weaned from the milk, and drawn from...**

***JEREMIAH 44:7*... child and suckling...**

***LAMENTATIONS 4:3, 4*... they give suck to their young ones...**

***JOEL 2:16*... and those that suck the breast...**

***HOSEA 1:8*... when she had weaned...**

***PSALMS 8:2;* Out of the mouth of babes and sucklings...**

***PSALMS 131:2*... as a child that is weaned of his mother...**

***MATTHEW 21:16*... same as Psalms 131:2**

***MARK 13:17*... to them that give suck in those days...**

***LUKE 21:23*... same as Mark 13:17**

Take TIME out of your day to encourage your heart, spirit, and mind. When you are feeling like you cannot continue breastfeeding your child, these scriptures will refuel your inner person. Second Timothy 2:15 says: "Study to show thyself approved unto God, a workman that needeth not be ashamed, rightly dividing the Word of truth." God's Word is your support! It will help you through discouraging times. Look to Jesus! He will be there with you.

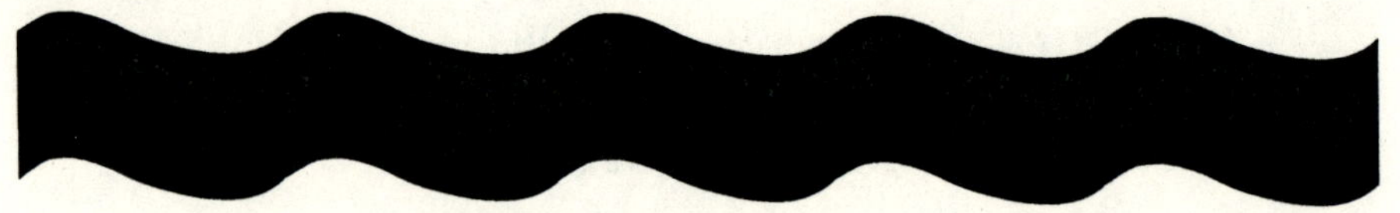

CHAPTER TWO

THE HISTORY OF MOTHERS WHO NURSED

At the turn of the century, nearly every baby was breast-fed by their mother or a wet nurse. If you do not know what wet-nurse means, let me explain. Wet-nursing is the complete nursing of another's infant, often for pay or when a mother was too ill to nurse her own child. In the Book of Exodus Chapter Two verses seven through ten in the Old Testament, written about 1250 B.C., tells of a wet-nurse being hired for Moses. (Unknown to her employer, the wet nurse was Moses' own mother!)[1] During the era of slavery in America, African-American mothers breast-fed their master's children when they were needed. In a few cases, white women breast-fed African-American children.[2]

---

[1] www.lalecheleague.org, wet-nursing
[2] www.greensboro.com, history of breastfeeding, p. 2

It was not until advances in sanitation, development of uncontaminated feeders, and significant alterations were made to cow's milk that artificial feeding became a possibility. Although most mothers assumed that the ingredients used to make baby formula are selected based on ingredients that provide nutrition, this is not the case.[3]

It was not until the early 1900's that mothers began to make a choice to nurse or not to nurse. Worldwide, babies are nursed for an average of 4.2 years.[4] Among some groups in other countries as many as ninety-five percent of mothers' breastfeed their babies.[5] People in America assume that even if you start out breastfeeding, you will soon wean your baby from the breast to the bottle. However, it is worth consideration to continue breastfeeding if your baby still has a need to suck or has a nutritional need for a high-fat, calorie-dense food (which babies do need until at least two years of age).[6]

Do you know because more and more mothers are now breastfeeding their babies, they are finding that they enjoy

---

[3] Compassionate Souls, p.27

[4] What to Expect When You're Expecting, p. 251-255

[5] A Doctor Discusses Nutrition During Pregnancy & Breast Feeding, p. 82

[6] Compassionate Souls, p. 27, 36-38

breastfeeding enough to want to continue longer than they initially thought? United Nations Children's Fund (UNICEF) has long encouraged breastfeeding for two years and longer, and the American Academy of Pediatrics is now on record as encouraging mothers to nurse at least one year or for as long as both mother and baby desire. Breastfeeding to three and four years of age has been common in much of the world until recently, and a breastfeeding toddler is still common in many societies.[7]

Nursing your baby is such a simple and natural process. Amazingly, it comes in a variety of flavors as a mother's diet varies. Breastfeeding is a process that you can treasure and have joy in doing because your baby is your gift from God. You and your baby were made for breastfeeding! From birth my baby was able to let me know when he was hungry. He was able to attach to my breast, to suck, swallow and digest my milk which was perfectly designed to meet his specific needs. God designed it that way for the mother and the baby. Just as it began with the first woman in the Bible so will He end it, no matter what society says or does? The scriptures prove that the

---

[7] Jane's Breastfeeding Resources: Breastfeeding Articles, p. 1

women of old did it God's way. However, we basically have not been taught this in the Body of Christ, or at home. Godly women should be teaching the younger, married women about the home and rearing their children. The scriptures instruct them to do so.

(Titus 2:3, 4 KJV) says:

> That the aged women likewise, that they be in behavior as becometh holiness, not false accusers, not given to much wine, teachers of good things; That they may teach the younger women to be sober, to love their husbands, to love their children,

---

In addition, these women with spiritual maturity knew their God and what He was capable of doing. God has not changed. He is the same yesterday, today, and, forever. They did not take thought as to whether they should or should not nurse their baby. This was not an option for them. I sincerely believe they knew for a certainty this would help the immune system of the baby. Because the immune system is crucial, the women of the Bible knew how long to nurse their baby and knew when it was time to wean the baby from the breast. Also, the husbands in the Bible seemed to be in agreement with the wife concerning the length of time to nurse and wean their child.

(I Samuel 1: 22-24, 27-28 KJV) says:

> But Hannah went not up; for she said unto her husband, I will not go up until the child be weaned, and then I will bring him, that he may appear before the LORD, and there abide forever.
>
> And Elkanah her husband said unto her, do what seemeth thee good; tarry until thou have weaned him; only the LORD establish his word. So, the woman abode, and gave her son, Samuel, suck until she weaned him.
>
> And when she had weaned him she took him up with her, with three bullocks, and one ephah of flour,

and a bottle of wine, and brought him unto the House of the LORD in Shiloh: and the child was young.

For this child I prayed; and the LORD hath given me my petition, which I asked of Him: Therefore also I have lent him to the LORD; as long as he liveth he shall be lent to the LORD. And he worshiped the LORD there.

(Exodus 2:9 KJV) says:

And Pharaoh's daughters said unto her, take this child away, and nurse it for me and I will give thee thy wages. And the woman took the child, and nursed it.

My study in the Scriptures concerning breastfeeding has been interesting as well as a blessing. We see in the scriptures, breastfeeding was a natural thing to do without question. The thought of not doing so would have been considered foolish. When the biological mother was unable to nurse the child, they found another mother who would be a wet nurse. This practice continued to happen during slavery times of my ancestors in America. Breastfeeding by the mother or wet nurse was still the only way to feed their newborn. Please take the time to educate yourself in the scriptures concerning the role of the women and mothers in the Bible. Educating yourself will be a theme continued throughout the book. The Bible is our ultimate life guide to teach us how to nurture our children.

(Luke 11:27 KJV) says:

And it came to pass, as he spake these things, a certain woman of the company lifted up her voice, and said unto him, Blessed is the womb that bare thee, and the paps which thou hast sucked.

(Genesis 49:25 KJV) says:

Even by the God of thy father, who shall help thee; and by the Almighty, who shall bless thee with blessings of heaven above, blessings of the deep that lieth under, blessings of the breasts, and of the womb:

You will not go wrong if you pray and follow God's instruction through your entire walk while living on the Earth.

When I first started breastfeeding, I committed to doing it for one year. When my son became a year old, it was apparent to me that breastfeeding was providing so much for him nutritionally and emotionally. Stopping at that point was out of the question, because of the sickle cell trait that he carry's. Breastfeeding during his early toddler stage was a wonderful way for him to calm down during church services or other outings. This became a time for us to bond with each other. Nursing him has continued to protect him from germs he was exposed to while playing with other children. The mother's milk is a protective substance against many illnesses such as colds, ear infections as well as stomach viruses. The child's immune system is greatly enhanced by the milk. This becomes a safety net for the child.

I find it interesting that anthropologists have studied other primates and have extracted data from their studies in an effort to determine the natural age for weaning a human child. They have estimated this to be near four to seven years of age. Until about the age of five, the saliva of most humans contains the enzyme lactase, which allows us to digest the lactose in milk.[8]

---

[8] Compassionate Souls, p. 39

In light of all the benefits of breastfeeding, I pray that my daughter, does it Gods way and breastfeeds her babies when that season comes for her to have a family. My desire for my son is for him to be an encouragement and support to his wife to nurse their babies.

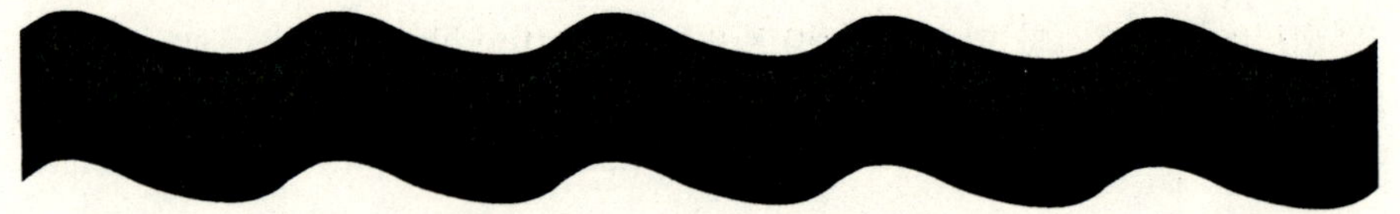

CHAPTER THREE

GIVING YOUR BODY & BABY THE BEST

In order to give your baby the best before, during, and after your pregnancy you must provide your body with the proper nutrients. It is important that you eat right. Good eating habits allow you to produce healthy milk for your baby. A breastfeeding mother needs to consume at least twenty-five hundred calories per day.[9] It is recommended that breastfeeding mothers consume slightly more nutrients than a mother who is not breastfeeding their baby.[10] Did you know that your body uses energy to produce your milk? It is the most nutritionally demanding time of your life. If you are not careful to replace the nutrients used to form your milk supply, your general health will

[9] Healthy Expectations, p. 216
[10] A Doctor Discusses Nutrition During Pregnancy & Breast Feeding, p. 84

eventually deteriorate. Provide your body and the baby's body with everything that is needed to prevent any common ailments and serious illnesses. Also, drink at least 10 glasses of water per day!

Just in case you do not receive your daily nutritional requirements through your foods, you may need to take quality, natural food supplements. I found them to be a tremendous benefit to my body.

Do to the way our food is grown and processed, we may not be getting our vitamin and mineral needs adequately met through what we eat. Farmers are using chemicals, herbicides, and pesticides. In addition the land is not allowed to rest for the replenishing of minerals.

By the time our fruits, vegetables, and meats are cooked and eaten, we have destroyed basically all of the vitamins and minerals we need for our body. In addition, sugar, artificial colorings, flavorings, and additives, are killing the natural enzymes in our body. Remember, our body is alive. We are living and breathing people created in the image of God. The purchase of organically grown produce may give you a slight edge over regularly grown produce. This is also true of organically fed livestock that we use as our meats.

I encourage you to do some research on a food supplement and find one you can trust and feel confident in taking. The quality and results are what you want to look for in supplements. I have been taking supplements along with eating properly for nine years; I noticed a big difference in my health. The supplements I take are of top quality ingredients and are pure concentrated food, not pills, drugs, or medicine. My personal preferences are the supplements made by the Shaklee Corporation.

I urge women to speak to their doctor and take a look at different supplements that are on the market. Even if you are not expecting a child or do not have children, some supplements can be good for you. Pray and asked the Lord to direct you to the right foods and supplements to take during the time you are pregnant and while you are nursing your baby.

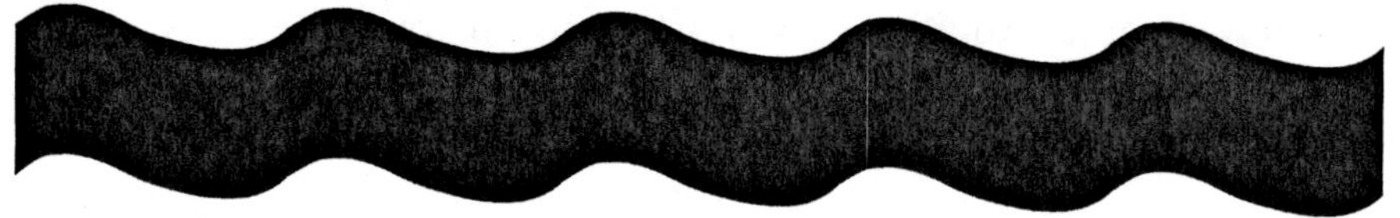

CHAPTER FOUR

MY DESIRE FOR SUPPORT

I wanted support from my family, friends, and others who would notice me breastfeeding. My understanding now is; in trying to get other people' support should not have been all that important when it came to making my decision. If you are not convinced on your own, then you will always be looking for others approval and support. Know for yourself that you want to breastfeed regardless if you receive the support you want or not. I received some encouragement from a very wise, older, woman in the Body of Christ. She never had anything negative to say regarding breastfeeding. She was very encouraging to me during some difficult times in my life. She would always speak words according to the scripture. Remember, God's word is spirit and life!

Many people would still continue to ask me questions about breastfeeding my son; “How do you do it?”; “Doesn’t it hurt?”; “Did he bit you yet?” Some would say, “There is no difference if you nursed or not”; others would say, “He is too big for you to continue nursing him.”; “If he can eat and talk he should not be nursing that long.”: It goes on and on with questions and negative statements. To say the least, there were no words of God’s love and encouragement from them.

Not receiving much support and encouragement from outsiders, since it is a natural thing to do after having a baby; I received all of the support I really needed from my husband. He was truly with me all the way through to the weaning stage. It is really all you need. Those who are married and have their husband’s support will have greater confidence and will probably nurse for a longer period of time.

The mindset of many people seems to be that nursing was only done during our grandmother’s time. Many believe it is not for this generation. They considered it to be old-fashioned. People say we now have technology to produce different types of formula to suit your child's need. Old-fashioned or not, it is still God's way; not how the women's movement has dictated it to be. The women's movement has gone against the Word God commands for married women. The women's movement exemplifies a freedom for woman that set their sights outside the nursery. Women wanted not only freedom but also control-control of their lives and control of their bodies. However, we know control was gained with knowledge. Gods' knowledge told them that nursing was best for their babies and, on the whole, for themselves. They knew this, yet some chose not to breastfeed regardless of knowledge presented to them. Ironically, the women's movement of the 1960's and 70's brought nursing back into vogue. Today, there is clearly a back to nursing trend.[11] Despite the numerous benefits of breastfeeding, the American Academy of Pediatrics notes that the numbers of mothers opting to breastfeed are still lower than expected: "Although breastfeeding rates have increased slightly since 1990, the percentage of women currently electing to breastfeed their babies is still lower than levels reported in the mid-1980s. "In 1995, it was determined by the AAP that 59.4

---

[11] What to Expect When You're Expecting, p. 251

percent of women in the United States were breastfeeding exclusively or in combination with formula-feeding at the time of hospital discharge. Only 21.6 percent of mothers were nursing at six months, and many of these were supplementing with formula."

Most women have too little information regarding the pros and benefits of breastfeeding and the dangers of artificial feeding to make a sound judgment. Because so many manufactures' advertisements and marketing ploys for baby formula, mothers are finding it difficult to make a choice to breastfeed.

According to the scriptures, it should be done no matter what picture the world paints if you desire to be a virtuous woman as **Proverbs 31:10 speaks of:**

"***Who can find a virtuous woman? For her price is far above rubies."***

Listen! Do you hear the Lord speaking to your heart? Know that God is trying to tell us something about our current life. We should listen to the Holy Spirit. Be that virtuous mother that God is speaking of!

Again, there are Biblical and medical facts to prove it. Do your own research and you will find plenty of documentation to support these words.

It has not been a hard thing to breastfeed in spite of my inadequacies. In obedience to and faith in what God told me to do for my son, I continued doing what I knew was right in my heart. Note; we hear through our ears and in our heart. I consider this a privilege to be able to nurse and give my son the very best of what God uniquely created to nourish his body for growth and development. Bear in mind mother's milk contains immunities to diseases and aids in the development of a baby's immune system.[12] This is very essential in a child's body. I am thankful to God that my son has not been sick as often as many of the children I know. Evidence shows that babies who are nursed are protected from common childhood illnesses such as colds, ear infections, and diarrhea during the early week and months of their life.[13]

I pray and encourage mothers to nurse their child if God gives you the opportunity, strength, and a sense of humor to breastfeed. Without

---

[12] 101 Reason to Breastfeed Your Child, number 10
[13] Compassionate Souls, p. 33; Baby Wise, p. 62

a doubt, you need strength and it only comes from God. Breastfeeding takes a lot of physical and emotional strength out of your body. You must drink plenty of water; eat enough calories to maintain your physical health and strength daily. Do not forget to read your Bible to maintain your spiritual strength to help you endure through this time of breastfeeding your baby.

(Psalm 73:26 KJV) says:

But GOD is the strength of my heart, and my portion forever.

(Proverbs 10:29 KJV) says:

The way of the LORD is strength to the upright:

American Academy of Pediatrics is urging mother's to nurse their baby for at least a year to six months, longer than previously advised.[14]

Do not let anyone discourage you from nursing your baby no matter what comments you hear! You must be confident in your own decision. When your mind is girded with the truth of Gods Word you will be able to stand strong even in the face of questions, stares, and negative remarks from others. Yet again, please educate yourself before you decide not to breastfeed so that there will not be any regrets.

(Proverbs 24:5 KJV) says:

A wise woman is strong, yea; a woman of knowledge increaseth strength.

Know that many mothers are not knowledgeable regarding nursing. Get knowledge from the Word of God. You will not go wrong. Knowledge is power. You need the power of God to equip you with His armor to defeat the attacks of the devil that may come through your decision to breastfeed your baby. We are to study to show ourselves approved by God. If you do not have the right data to

[14] Chicago (Associated Press) by Lindsay Tanner

back up what you are saying or doing, people will basically not take you or your information seriously. They may see you as a joke!

***(Hosea 4:6 KJV)* says:**

> My people are destroyed for lack of knowledge: because thou hast rejected knowledge, I will also reject thee, that thou shalt be not a priest to me: seeing thou hast forgotten the law of thy GOD, I will also forget thy children.

There is much information to be obtained about nursing your child. Invest in the time for you to acquire the knowledge you need to explain to those who ask, "Why do you nurse your baby?" When you give an answer, it should be powerful and stated with authority and love. When answering someone's question always answer in love and not defensively! Mother's do not have to be people pleasers. Your soul desire should be to just please God. He is the only One to have the final say regarding the life decisions made pertaining to your children. Continue to do what God tells you to do for your children no matter what negative thoughts or doubts come your way.

(Proverbs 3:6 KJV) says:

In all thy ways acknowledge him, and he shall direct thy paths.

Contact the La Leche League at 1(800) LA LECHE or look at their website[15], check out ProMom Inc.[16], and American Academy of Pediatrics on Breastfeeding and the use of Human Milk websites, if you need additional information. I recommend you become involved with several support groups. Talk to your pediatrician about information he or she may have available concerning breastfeeding. This can help you stay confident and motivated to nurse or continue nursing your child for a longer period of time.

[15] www.lalecheleague.org
[16] www.promom.org

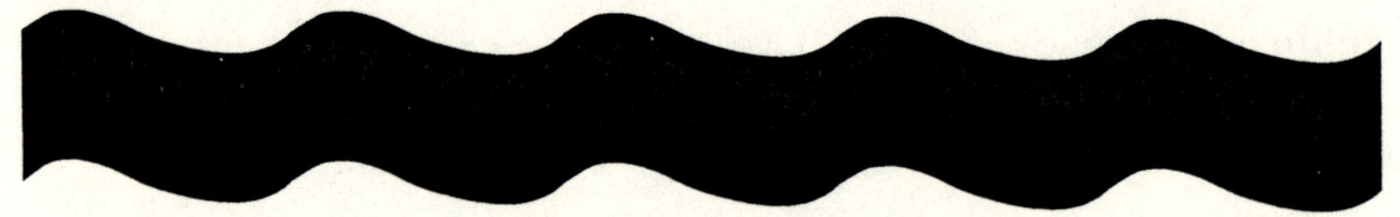

CHAPTER FIVE

NURSING YOUR BABY

I encourage, edify, and exhort all mothers' who are presently nursing their babies to continue to nurse regardless of the companies who work so hard to make bottle-feeding the norm with all the skillful marketing ploys that they use. The companies say that bottle-feeding is superior and more modern than breastfeeding. Nevertheless, breastfeeding gives your precious ones a loving foundation for a healthy life. You will be doing the right thing for your child and have the satisfaction of knowing that you are enriching both your baby's life and your own.

Many medical professionals have collaborated together in order to change the way society views breastfeeding. Lured by the desire to standardize and control nursing, they try to give a space for legitimacy.[17] Many doctors have been offered research grants and gifts in exchange for distributing free formula samples to their patients instead of suggesting breastfeeding. In addition, formula companies have hired women with the appearance of being a nurse to visit new mothers in the hospital. They also make home visits to new mothers. Wearing their nurses' uniform, they are being paid commissions that exceed the usual pay received by nurses. This is all in an effort to convince a mother not to breastfeed their infant. These women are often mistaken for hospital personnel. They gain access to new mothers in order to promote artificial milk as superior to breast milk.[18] According to the book, Milk, Money, and Madness by Naomi Baumslag M.D., formula sales have tripled over the past ten years and the industry is now bigger than ever, generating an astounding twenty–two million dollars every day in revenues. Suddenly, a new disease called Insufficient Milk Syndrome has been diagnosed, as mothers increasingly come to believe they are not capable of producing adequate milk for their baby.[19] Know that you are capable of producing enough milk for your baby if you trust the Lord and take

[17] Compassionate Souls, p. 28
[18] Compassionate Souls, p. 28

care of your body. Do not be deceived by the lies from the devil and the companies he uses to promote his scheme!

By the many negative comments I have heard and by the efforts of the formula companies, one can see that it is not the "in thing" to breastfeed your child. Nevertheless, if you decide to breastfeed, you are doing it God's way in that He decided to produce milk from inside a woman's breast to feed her baby. Being able to do nurse an infant is designed and ordained by the Almighty Creator, God. As we should know, He is the One who created our physical body.

As I approached my delivery date, I told the Lord, "If He would give me the courage and strength to nurse my son, I would do so." The many unpleasant stories told to me by other mothers caused me to doubt my ability to nurse. Some of these stories were "It is so inconvenient!"; "It hurts your breast!"; "I do not have time to pump my breast; I just can not do it!" I almost allowed this to sabotage my thinking towards breastfeeding. However, I wanted to nurse my baby. I knew in my heart that it was right for me and it was God's way. God gave me my breasts with milk that produces a substance that softens

---

[19] Compassionate Souls, p. 30

the baby's skin. This same substance can be used as a healing ointment when the nipple is sore. This is done by squeezing a small amount of milk from the breast and rubbing it on the sore nipple. This same substance may also slow the growth of bacteria. The scent of this substance is what guided my son to my breast for nourishment during his infancy. I continued to pray and to nurse as long as God directed me to do so and it left me with such a peace regarding my decision.

Breastfeeding is far more than just sustenance for the infant. I have found the mother-infant bonding to be a great benefit. After having two C-sections, I experienced post-partum depression. Breastfeeding was a mental healing for me. It has been a great source of comfort to my son and my daughter and as you can see for myself.

When the nurse brought my son to me for his first feeding, he latched on to my breast immediately without any problem. The certified lactation nurse who was helping me stated, "I have never seen this happen in all of the twenty years of being a consultant." Truly, I count it a blessing from The Most High God to have been able to nurse initially with no problems. The only discomfort I felt was my uterus contracting. However, it lasted for only a short time. Nursing helps your womb to return to normal, so it is not unusual to feel your uterus tightening while you are feeding your baby. I continued to educate myself about breastfeeding and all of the wonderful things that happens when you do.

Continuing to nurse, I made a commitment to God and my husband to nurse him for at least a year. During this time my son went through growth spurts, which is normal for a baby.

I produced so much milk! The milk would come in so well. It seemed as though I was being milked like a cow! Sometimes it would just squirt all over his face. My son would empty both breast within eight to ten minutes and then go to sleep for three to four hours. It was great that he would sleep that long. I was able to do things around the house or take a nap.

I noticed how alert and healthy my son was, which I attributed to breastfeeding. His skin had a bright glow and it was smooth and clear. Ear infections were not a problem with him as it is with so many babies. I did not have many doctor visits as a result of him not being sick. To confirm factually why he was doing so well, I began reading everything I could about breastfeeding. I would spend many hours of studying the subject of nursing to confirm what God had ordained. While studying, I discovered why mother's milk is the very best and that nothing can compare to it! I mean absolutely nothing!!!! Nothing being produce can begin to come close to it! Research has proven that breastfeeding stimulates the infant immune system. The mother's milk contains numerous other factors of likely significance for the defense of the infant. For example, a mother's milk provides perfect infant nutrition.[20] The milk also provides valuable omega-3 fatty acids that protect the body and even improves the IQ of the baby.[21] In addition, it decreases the risk of dying from respiratory infection by 3.6 fold compared with formula or cow's milk feeding.[22] There are numerous written studies on breastfeeding that encourage a mother to nurse her infant without anxiety regarding what people may imply. John McDonald M.D., author of a number of books on health and the practice of medicine, minces no words when he talks about the

---

[20] 101 Reasons to Breastfeed Your Child, number 4
[21] Healthy Expectations, p. 215
[22] Breastfeeding Stimulates the Infant Immune System, p. 8

importance of breastfeeding. He feels it is practically child abuse to deprive your infant of your milk.[23]

Medical scientists have been trying for years to duplicate the mother's milk. They cannot! No one can top that which is from the Creator God. Only The God of Heaven and Earth can create milk in a woman's breast to nurture her infant properly. The mother's milk always has the right proportions of fat, carbohydrates, and protein. How awesome it is that you can give your baby a full course meal all at once, always at the right temperature. Wow, isn't that amazing!

Formula companies are constantly adjusting these proportions looking for the best composition. You see, man is trying to take the place of God and do that which only God can do. He will never be able to accomplish this. God knew that it could never be matched. The mother's milk composition changes from feeding to feeding depending on the needs of her child.[24] Increasingly, researchers have begun to clearly demonstrate that mother's milk is the best food for your baby.[25]

---

[23] Compassionate Soul, p. 33
[24] 101 Reason to Breastfeed Your Child, number 51
[25] A Doctor Discusses Nutrition During Pregnancy & Breast Feeding, p. 81

In my tenth month I prayed and asked God if I should stop. In my spirit, the Lord answered me and said no, "continue on". Because of what people would say, I continued to pray about breastfeeding and received a peace in my spirit to continue for one more year. Nursing past six months basically is unheard of in this generation. I sensed God giving me such a peace in my heart and mind that He would naturally wean my child from my breast. While nursing him, I would always tell my son that he would be weaned by the time he was two years old. I would tell him this every time I would nurse him. I received an instruction kit from my Lamaze class on weaning, which assisted me in the process. Studies have shown that after weaning your baby, breastfed infants have lowered risk of dying from infections.[26] Most of the world knows there are so many diseases and infections that babies can acquire. It is good to know that breastfeeding my child will help reduce the many probabilities regarding disease.

As a mother who genuinely believes in nursing her child, I wholeheartedly advocate breastfeeding. I want to communicate

---

[26] Breastfeeding Stimulates the Infant Immune System, p. 8

plainly and truthfully to all mothers the importance of giving your baby this gift of love given by God. I encourage you Biblically and on a factual basis as well. Literally, some doctors try to convince their patients that it is best health wise for the mother as well as the baby.[27] A large study showed that each month of breastfeeding decreases infant mortality by 6.2 per one thousand.[28]

Everything in my natural life is parallel to my spiritual life. God desires us to be in good health even as our souls prosper. If you are not physically healthy, your soul will not be spiritually healthy because there is a lack of God's word working in your life.

(3 John 1:2 KJV) says:

> Beloved, I wish above all things that though mayest prosper and be in health, even as thy soul prosperth.

A new mother would be wise to take heed to honest, sound research, and what the scriptures have to say about breastfeeding. Do

[27] A Doctor Discusses Pregnancy, p. 107

not be just a reader of God's word, but be a doer of His Word. Do not allow your mind to talk you out of a healthy blessing that is beneficial for your baby and your body as well.

Initially you may feel uncomfortable breastfeeding around people. Do not permit this to hinder your efforts. You should always make sure that the feeding is done discreetly and modestly. There is always the option of using another room, your automobile, or sitting away from those around you for more privacy. You should choose what makes you feel comfortable. Of course, if you still are not sure about nursing your baby in public, there are maternity stores that sell nursing wear and bras. These are designed for convenience to cover the infant and the mothers' breast and to make her feel comfortable and confident. Also you can use larger tops or your husband's shirts if you can't afford the cost of nursing wear. Where there is a will, there is a way.

With the help of the Lord, you can breastfeed your baby successfully. I did it with confidence and assurance because of His

---

[28] Breastfeeding Stimulates the Infant Immune System, p. 8

guidance. First pray, make the commitment, and then educate yourself about breastfeeding. You must be persistent in your endeavor.

You can be educated about breastfeeding by attending La Leche League meetings prior to giving birth. The La Leche League is a source of information and support for a full range of mothering–related issues. This league was founded in 1956 by a group of seven nursing mothers. They were concerned that breastfeeding rates in the United States had dropped to around twenty percent of new mothers. There are over three thousand local groups in the United States, which operates a twenty-four-hour help line. They offer extensive literature covering a wide range of topics related to better mothering through breastfeeding.

For more information about the League call your lactation consultant from your hospital help line, if available. This information helps you to make an informed decision even though you may not be planning to breastfeed your baby. Ask your doctor or midwife as many questions as you can, pertaining to breastfeeding. Your public library can be a wealth of information on this subject. It is very important to educate yourself. I cannot emphasize the importance of this enough. Do your research early on! Read all of the breastfeeding magazines, pamphlets, handouts, books, and call friends who are knowledgeable and can offer their input.

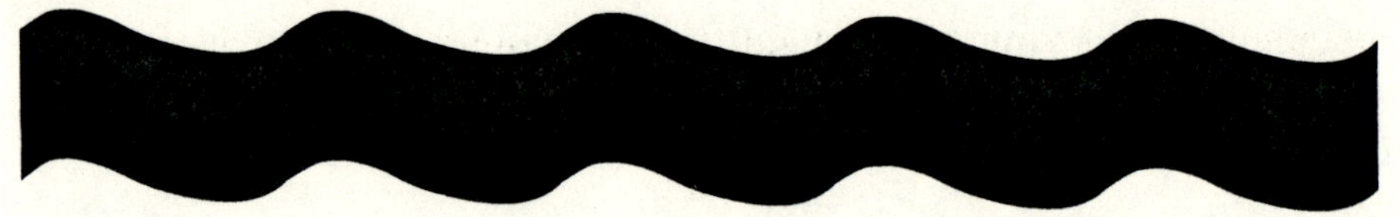

CHAPTER SIX

FOR A SEASON

Breastfeeding is absolutely the optimum food for the baby during this period of time in their life. If my baby was being nursed whenever they desired, there is no need to give my child anything else the entire first year. For example, I do not observe animals coming to humans to nurse their young. Animals nurse their own young completely without introducing another animal's milk. If we are God's highest creation on the Earth, why do we give our baby cow's milk or any other milk other than our own for a least one-year.

In my twenty-one months of nursing my son, the time was great. Breastfeeding was an awesome experience to be able to nurse for this length of time. My son is alert, energetic, fun, intelligent, and social. As my son is growing older and healthier, it is amazing seeing this happening before my eyes. I do have to continue to eat healthy in order to maintain a good milk flow. I am conscious of what I eat and my health is being sustained.

My son began weaning himself from the breast as his desire to nurse decreased from how it was initially.

When we read the Scriptures we are told about nursing and weaning our children. Now the question is raised, how long were children nursed in Biblical times? In the Eastern part of the world, weaning is often deferred for as long as three years.[29] If we look in Exodus Chapter Two, Moses was three months old when his mother set him adrift down the Nile River as seen in verse two. However, in verses seven through nine it is apparent that he was not yet weaned. Pharoah's daughter unknowingly hired Moses' mother (Jochebed, Exodus 6:20) to be his wet-nurse, and so he was breastfed well beyond three months. In verse ten, we are told that the child grew. Clearly, the period of time that Jochebed nursed her son for the Pharoah's daughter was longer than just a few months. According to a rabbinic commentary, it says that Moses was two years old at the

[29] The Zondervan Pictorial Bible Dictionary, p. 888

point of his weaning and adoption by the princess of Egypt.[30] As mentioned earlier in the passage of First Samuel Chapter One, gives me some indication as to the age of Hannah weaning her son. Hannah weaned Samuel before she dedicated him to a life of service in the Tabernacle where she prayed and vowed in Shiloh for him. Bible scholars agree that the age at which Hannah weaned Samuel was more like three years of age.[31] Overall, the Biblical evidence presented here does not actually tell us when children were weaned from the breast. Nevertheless, these Scriptural references certainly lead us to the conclusion that in Biblical times children were breastfed for a substantial length of time, a time frame measured not in months but in years.[32]

In this generation, breastfeeding is considered absurd if you go past six months. Personally, I knew that God would give me the strength to wean my son by his second birthday. Now, his life must enter the next season of his growth and development. The day that my son was weaned, my husband and I had a celebratory feast (went to

---

[30] www.texas-midwife.com/breastfeeding, p.1-5

[31] www.texas-midwife.com/breastfeeding, (Clarke, Vol. 1, p.133; McClintock & Strong, Vol. X, p. 892)

[32] www.texas-midwife.com/breastfeeding, p. 7

dine at a restaurant) and an offering of thanks to God for everything that transpired during this season of our lives.

(Genesis 21:8 KJV) says:

> And the child grew, and was weaned: and Abraham made a great feast the same day that Isaac was weaned.

When you do what God says, there will be great results. He will continue to bless you in your obedience. As stated earlier, everything that is contained in the scriptures is parallel in the natural realm. For instance, as He desires for baby's to have their mother's milk, He also desires for us to have the sincere milk of the Word when we are babes in Christ. When you are a newborn baby, you are unable to eat meat and digest it properly! You must begin with what you are able to handle. For the baby that is breast milk.

(1 Peter 2:2 KJV) says:

As newborn babes, desire the sincere milk of the word that ye may grow thereby:

God nourishes us through His Word so that we can flourish in the things pertaining to our life. You can be assured by Gods Word that He knows what is best in everything that concerns us. He wants to protect the mothers and their children from the attack of the devil when it comes to diseases and sicknesses in their bodies.

Here are Several Reasons why God wants to protect our babies and ourselves:

- **A study of women in rural China found that not nursing increases mother's risk of breast cancer: women who breast fed their babies for two years or longer reduced their risk of breast cancer by 50%.**[33]
- **Protects against infection in industrialized countries** [34]

---

[33] The Plain Dealer, Cleveland, Ohio, 1/31/01

[34] Breastfeeding Stimulates Infant Immune System, p. 8

- **Nursing helps the baby pass me conium (baby bowel movement)**
- **Nursing helps prevent post-partum hemorrhage**
- **Protects against anemia**
- **Protects against Crohn's disease**
- **Decreases insulin requirements for moms**
- **Stabilizes progress of maternal endometriosis**
- **Nursing decreases mom's risk of developing ovarian cancer**
- **Lowers risk of baby developing asthma**
- **Protects against bacterial meningitis in infants**
- **Protects against respiratory infections**
- **Protects baby against vision defects**
- **Is an intestinal soother for the baby**
- **Is a natural contraceptive-helps space your children depending on how you breastfeed**
- **Natural pain relief for baby and an antibiotic for wounds** [35]

[35] 101 Reasons to Breastfeed Your Child

- **Cut in half the incidence of diarrhea**
- **Urinary tract infections are less common**
- **The World Health Organization has indicated that increasing breastfeeding by 40% would reduce respiratory deaths by 50% and diarrhea deaths by 66% worldwide in children less than eighteen months of age.**
- **Study among a large group of Finnish children found that breastfeeding for more than one month resulted in significant reductions in food allergy at years one to three and asthma up to age seventeen.**
- **Several studies investigated the protective capacity of breastfeeding against allergy, avoiding common food allergens in the diet of lactating mothers in families with a high risk of allergy decreases the prevalence of topic dermatitis.**
- **Protects against wheezing, bronchitis for six to seven years.**[36]

---

[36] Breastfeeding Stimulates Infant Immune System, p. 7-9

- *Sudden Infant Death Syndrome (SIDS) - a study indicated that breastfeeding was protective against SIDS, consistent with an effect mediated through the prevention of gastrointestinal and/or respiratory disease* [37]
- *Not breastfeeding at discharge from an obstetric hospital at any stage of the infants' life was associated with an increased risk of SIDS.* [38]
- *A protection against pollution: With increasing level of pollution and contamination that is pervasive in our environment and present to some extent in all plants and animals-even those raised organically –many mothers are concerned about how they can reduce the level of pesticides and endocrine-disrupting chemicals in their milk. According to a letter printed in The England*

---

[37] Hoffman, H.J., Risk Factors for SIDS: Results of the National Institute of Child Health and Human Development SIDS Cooperative Epidemiological Study. Ann NY ACAD Science, 1988

Journal of Medicine on March 26, 1981, researchers found that the breast milk of women whose diets were composed exclusively of plants had only one to two percent of the level of various chemicals found in the milk of the average American women. Another study published in 1983 in the Scandinavian medical journal Acta Paediatr Scand showed that women who didn't eat meat but drank cow's milk had lower levels of contaminants in their milk than omnivores. Women who consumed a lot of fish had milk that was the most polluted. (This makes sense since the fish humans eat are the final link in the food chain.) [39]

- *It improves neurological development.*[40]
- *It is good for the environment such as there is not plastic containers..*

The Maternal Benefits:[41]

---

[38] Mitchell, A. "Results from the First Year of the New Zealand Count Death Study". N.Z. Med A, 1991; 104:71-76

[39] Compassionate Souls, p. 39

- It benefits the mother's health
- Delays fertility (women who nurse frequently during exclusive breastfeeding remained amenorrhoeic (free from menses) longer than infrequent nursers, supplements introduced later and did not resume menses as promptly thereafter. Duration of exclusive nursing and night nursing after supplementation were the major influences on amenorhoea) [42]

Decreases

- Breast Cancer
- Uterine Cancer
- Ovarian Cancer
- Endometrial Cancer
- Emotional Health
- Insulin Requirements

---

[40] Compassionate Souls, p. 39
[41]www.breastfeeding.com
[42] Elias, M.F. "Nursing Practices and Lactation Amenorrhoea" Journal of Biosco Science, 1968

- Osteoporosis
- Promote Postpartum Weight Loss

Societal Benefits: [43]

- Optimum Child Spacing
- Improved Vaccine Effectiveness
- Financial Savings to Government and Families (food expenses, medical expenses)
- More Ecological
- Less Child Abuse

First and foremost the main benefit of breastfeeding is watching your happy, healthy child grow up; knowing you have given your infant the very best you can give as a mother. Do you see how God is wise enough to know how all these things would benefit our bodies overall?

(James 1:5 KJV) says:

[43] www.breastfeeding.com (jonahr@netins.net)

If any of you lack wisdom, let him ask of GOD, that giveth to all men/women liberally, and upbraideth not; it shall be given him/her.

By no means should you forget that God takes us through seasons for everything in life.

(Ecclesiastes 3:1 KJV) says:

To everything there is a season, and a time to every purpose under the heavens:

Recognize your season for your children and your household, because breastfeeding is not something you have to do forever. This is really a short portion of time out of your life here on this planet called Earth. Nonetheless, it is very important to know what you do, and why you do what you do regarding the life of your children.

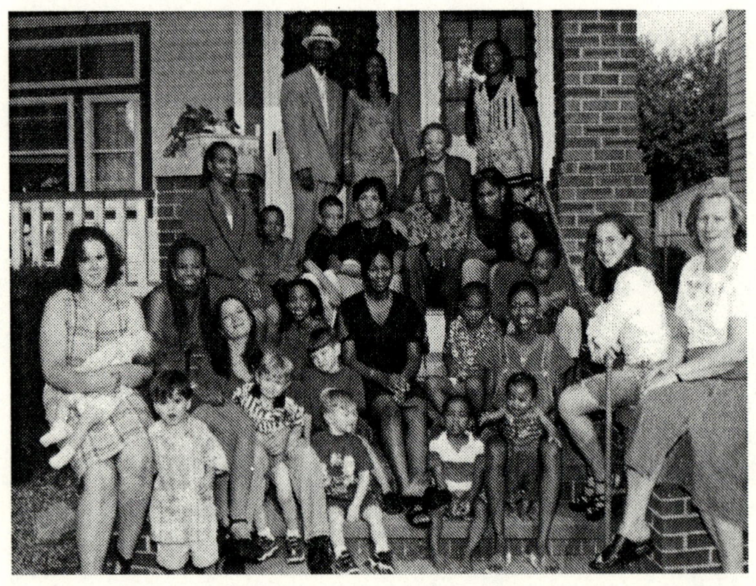

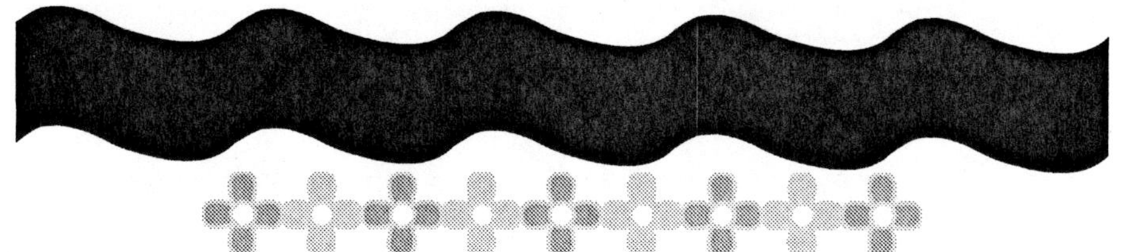

CHAPTER SEVEN

TESTIMONIES

MOTHERS, who are nursing their baby, have nursed or are "planning to nurse"

"All of these mothers have a different testimony that will speak to you wherever your heart and mind may be regarding breastfeeding your infant. I pray that these words impact your decision as a mother who desires to breastfeed." These mothers come from various backgrounds and cultures. I pray you will be blessed as you read each woman's testimony:

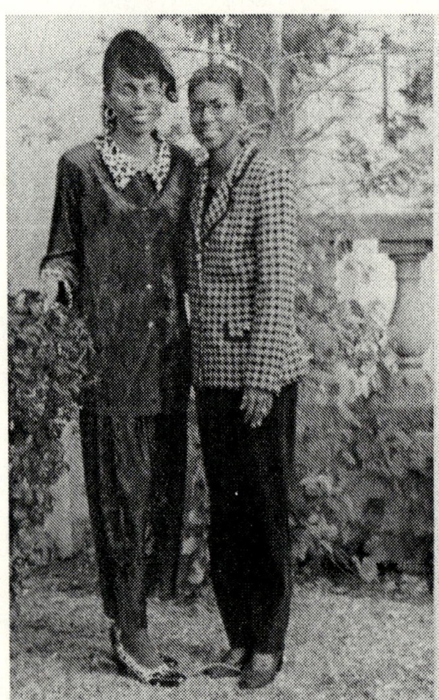

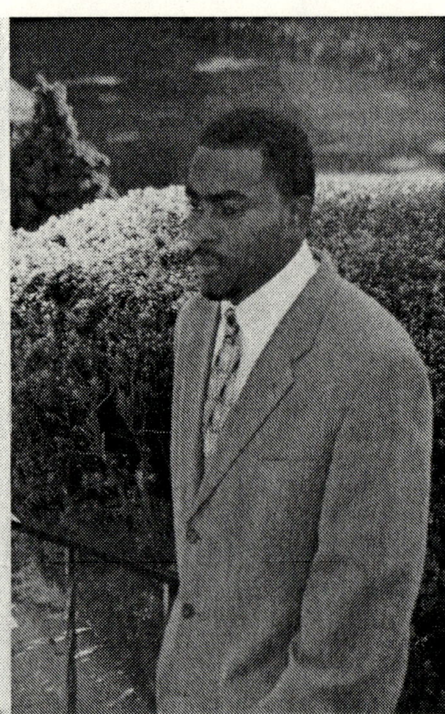

JoAnn M. Davis (Cleveland, Ohio)
My mother of 3 Children:
Gwendolyn-32; Melvin Jr.-30, Thaddaus-25
youngest son not pictured

My mother:

JoAnn M. Davis, *mother of 3 children – 32, 30, 25 (Cleveland, OH) Age: 53*

Person of Color

In 1970, I did not breastfeed my daughter, Gwen. During my pregnancy I developed a bronchial condition and this would not allow me to breastfeed. At that time I did not understand the many positive reasons about breastfeeding. I had to use store bought formula.

In 1972, I had my second child, Melvin, Jr. Melvin was born in my seventh month (approximately two pounds and three ounces). He was delivered by C-section. He was sickly and had to be confined to an incubator for about a month. I was not aware that I could breastfeed him. Again, I used the formula method.

In 1977 my youngest son, Thaddaus, was delivered by C-section also. I decided to breastfeed him because he was eight pounds and an active baby. He had a good appetite. I breast fed him for about three months and began again using formula because I had to return to work. Had I known what I know today, I feel that I would have done things differently. It is important that mothers obtain the right nutrition for a healthy body. I found it to be convenient and a wonderful experience. While breastfeeding my son, I started to understand how close a mother can be to her child emotionally. As a woman in the Body of Christ, it is important that all mothers breastfeed since it was ordained by God. I felt that I was cheated in the process.

I am very proud of Gwen's determination to breastfeed her children and the proper procedures she has taken in encouraging mothers to breastfeed their children."

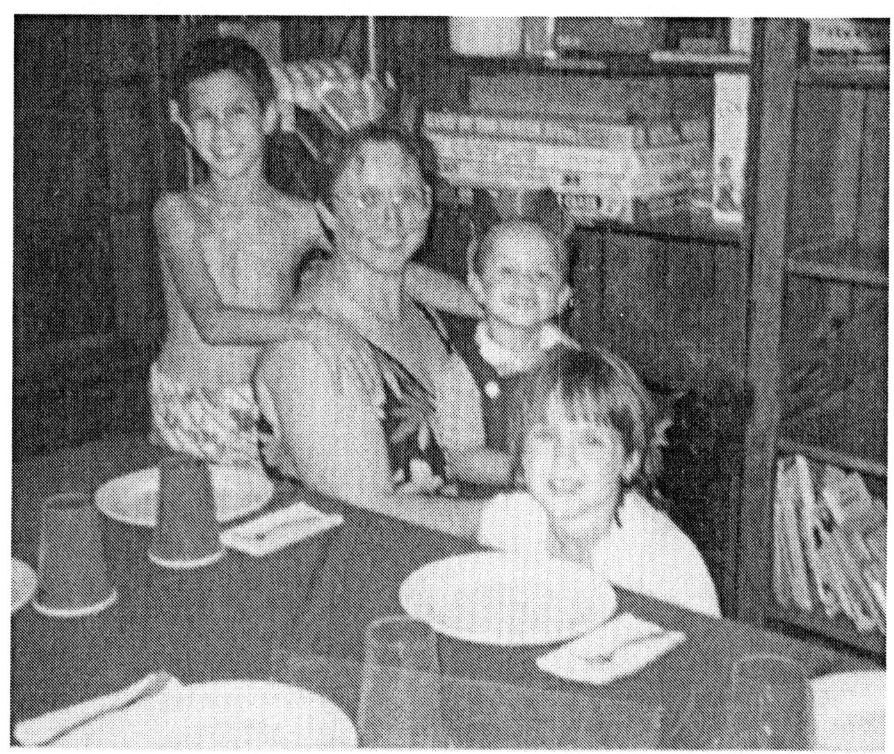

Marta Bruckman (Cleveland, Ohio)
Mother of 3 children:
Andrew Joseph-22; Emily Marie-20; Benjamin Joseph-17

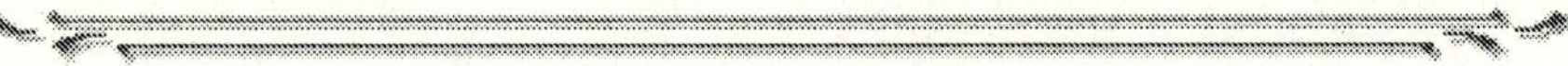

Marta Bruckman, *mother of 3 children – 22, 20, 17 (Cleveland, OH) Age: 53*

Hungarian

"For the first four months each of my children was breastfeed exclusively. Breastfeeding was the natural thing to do. I had heard that it was good to breastfeed because the mother passes on natural immunities to her child. However, my pediatrician left the decision to breastfeed totally up to me.

My husband was very supportive. He agreed with all the positive points for breastfeeding. He would help me by getting a blanket and keeping me covered while I nursed in public.

It was less expensive and handy to breastfeed. There were no bottles to wash, sterilize, and no formula to fuss with. I had been told how wonderful breastfeeding was and I wanted to have that experience.

My mother breastfed me also. It was what all mothers did in Europe.

I did not become engorged and I did not have to go through a painful drying up period. Breastfeeding helps to bring the uterus back to normal size more quickly.

Breastfeeding was a benefit to my baby. The benefits to my babies were that my milk immunities were passed on to him/her. My initial milk or colostrums was especially rich in a higher amount of fat and protein. I know that a human baby is much better off drinking human mother's milk rather than cow's milk. I feel that my children had fewer health problems than others who were bottle fed.

At four months, with each child, I was forced to take medications that would be passed through the milk to the child and I had to wean them "cold turkey". This was a heart-wrenching experience and very traumatic to me. I had no options. Nevertheless, they each took to the bottle very well.

Breastfeeding was physically enjoyable. It is a great release of pressure. Just being the supplier of your child's nourishment is a great joy. The child comes to know you as that supplier and looks to you for nourishment. There is a great bonding, closeness and love between mother and child.

I would and do encourage moms to breastfeed. I would simply say to you (mom) that God provided all the "equipment" and supplies all the milk. Why not take advantage of that. One of God's Hebrew names is the "Breasted One".—meaning that He is the supplier of everything we need. A mother is the supplier of everything an infant needs for up to the first full year of his/her life."

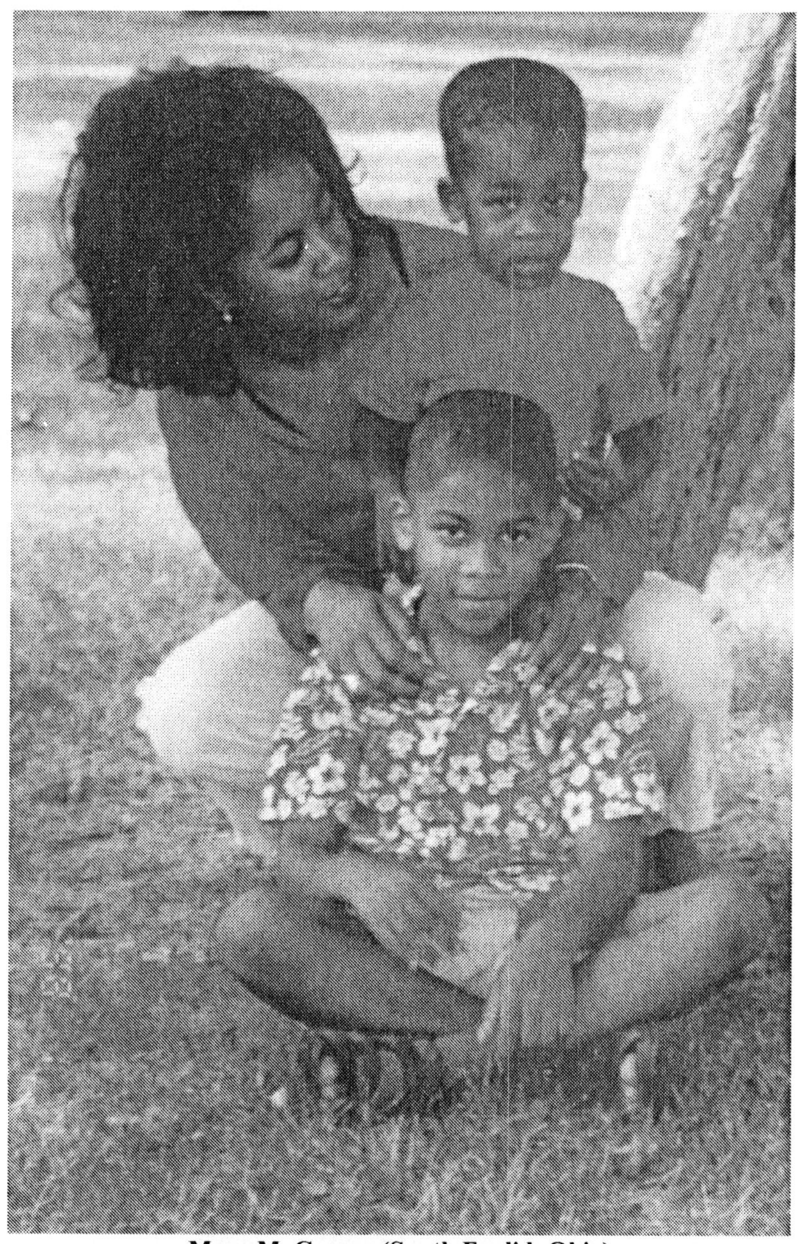

Myra M. George (South Euclid, Ohio)
Mother of 2 boys:
Joshua-5; Jordan-22 months

Myra Michele George, *mother of 2 boys – 5, 22 months (South Euclid, OH) Age: 34*

Person of color

"I decided to breastfeed my first son in 1996. Unfortunately my son had to be admitted at birth to the intensive care unit. I was introduced to him twelve hours later. When I went to him, the nurses informed me that my son was on Isomil infant formula! I remember feeling slighted and angry that no one had asked my permission.

My impending return to the workplace neared and I started supplementation along with breastfeeding. This entailed a lot of work! Bottles, nipples, sterilizing, sore breasts, and leakage…the feeding cycle seemed never-ending! During this time, I had to leave my baby for three, three-week sessions in another state! This was difficult emotionally as well as physically. You can imagine my distress at having to leave my infant so young and helpless. Physically, I tried to maintain the pumping morning and night in my hotel room. I had to endure leaking nipples during meetings, surges of pain and soreness throughout my breasts. My breast enlarged to the size of grapefruits. This was a constant reminder that my baby needed me as much as I needed him. I stopped the whole process of breastfeeding after 6 months.

Four years later, my second son arrived and I was resolved to strictly breastfeeding. I was confident in my position as a mother, assertive in my decision, and adamant against the filthy high price of formula. As I left the workforce to raise my sons, I had resolved to do the best for my children; and the best was breastfeeding. I breast fed my son for 14 months. He quickly found my breast and sucked from it.

He turned a year old, and I was still nursing him. It is important that we wean the children properly because at times I wish that I could recapture one more of those precious moments of closeness, kissing his skin, and remembering the smell of his hair."

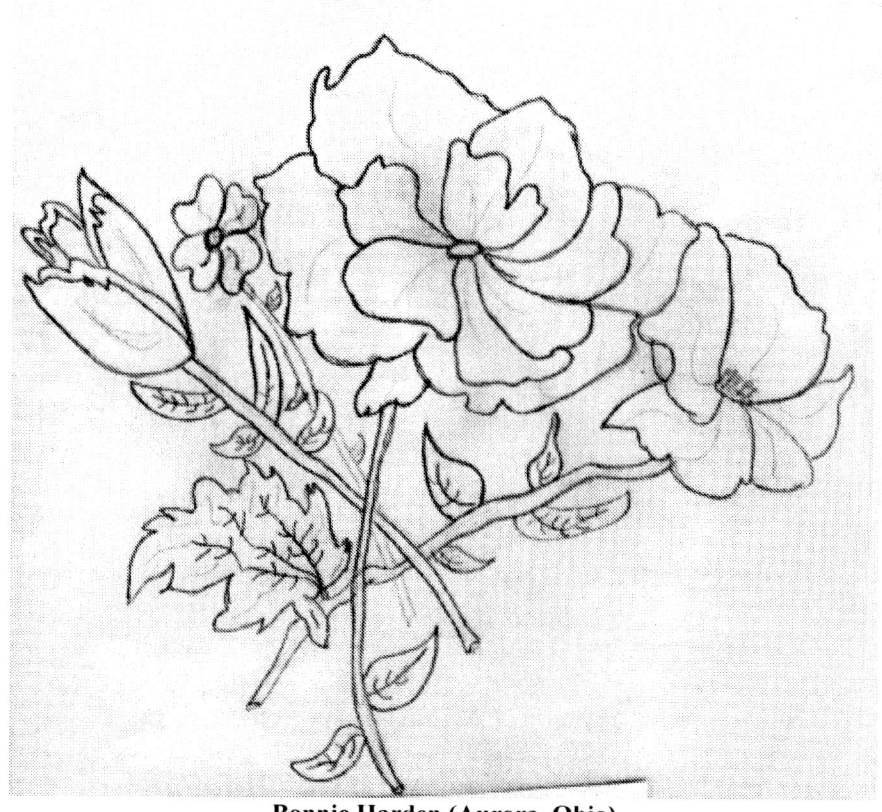

Bonnie Harden (Aurora, Ohio)
Expecting mother, due date April, 2003

Bonnie Harden, *expecting 17 weeks in the womb (Aurora, OH)*

Age: 28

Jewish

"I would like to breastfed because it is the best option and more importantly my doctor, who is a male, asked me if I was going to nurse. He said he was very happy to hear that I was planning to do this because it is the best for the baby and me. In reading, I found that the negatives of breastfeeding were cosmetic and did not find a lot of medical reasons for not breastfeeding. I do not fit in the cosmetic view of this society; it does not apply to me. In Judaism there is a saying, "Do the best by your child and you are a mother the day you conceive".

My mother did not breastfed me. She could not produce enough milk to breastfeed."

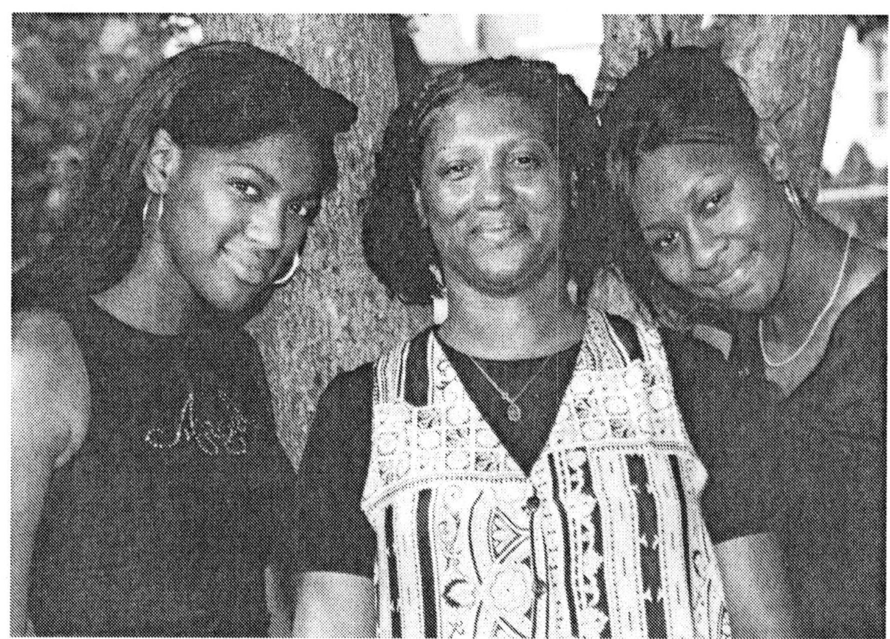

Cheryl Holloway (Euclid, Ohio)
Mother of three children:
Keanna-18; Michael-17; Octavia-16
son not pictured

Cheryl Holloway, *mother of 3 children -18, 17, 16 (Euclid, OH)*

Age: 41

Person of color

"As a mother of three children, I chose to nurse all of them. I believe nursing my children brought a close bond between us. My children were very healthy with few illnesses. I credit breastfeeding. I believe nursing is God-given. God equipped the woman's body with what the baby needs. I highly recommend nursing to any new mother."

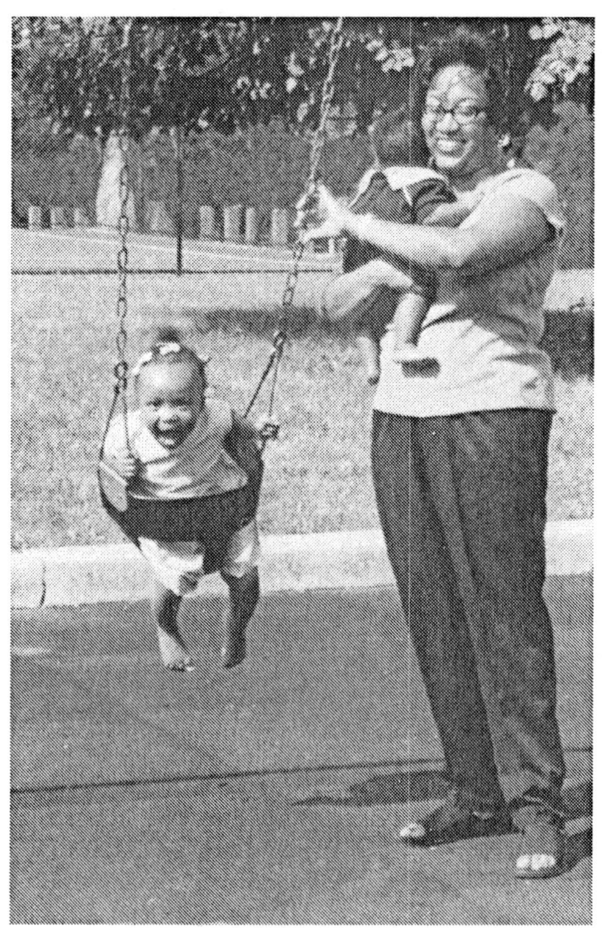

Charlotte Laird (Cleveland, Ohio)
Mother of a girl and boy:
Zipporah-1 ½; Shemah-2 months

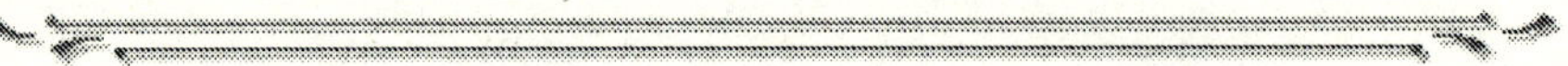

Charlotte Laird, *mother of 2 children -- 1 ½, 2 months (Cleveland, OH) Age: 30*

Person of color

"During my pregnancy I had planned to nurse. Several nurses began telling me the different positions for breastfeeding after I had the baby. Each nurse had her own preference as how to breastfeed. I became confused and frustrated. However, I still nursed the best way I knew how using the information that each nurse had given me.

One nurse in particular saw my determination to breastfeed and was willing to augment the feeding by taping tube-like syringes to my breast close to the nipple when it was time to feed. This allowed the baby to suck at the nipple and receive nourishment through the tube. This caused a sucking action to stimulate the milk flow. I was still frustrated with the process of breastfeeding, but in my heart I did not want to quit. I was still doing the syringe procedure until I had peace about stopping and my baby was able to latch on.

I felt that I would be doing my daughter a disservice if I did not nurse her. I would talk to my friend often and she would encourage me and tell me that she was praying for me. I believe because of my diligence in praying to God, it just became clear and easy to me. I nursed my daughter because I knew that it was healthy for her. I really enjoyed it and it brought forth a great bond between us. I nursed her a little over a year. I believe that God intended for mothers to breastfeed their child.

Nursing now was easy for me as well as a blessing because I had great support from my husband. I have seen great results from nursing, such as: her skin being smooth and clear, she was healthy, and was not sickly during the cold season.

With my son, he latched on with no problem. Now I am a pro at breastfeeding and I can actually teach other moms. Supplementation with Shaklee vitamins was very important during my pregnancy and while nursing."

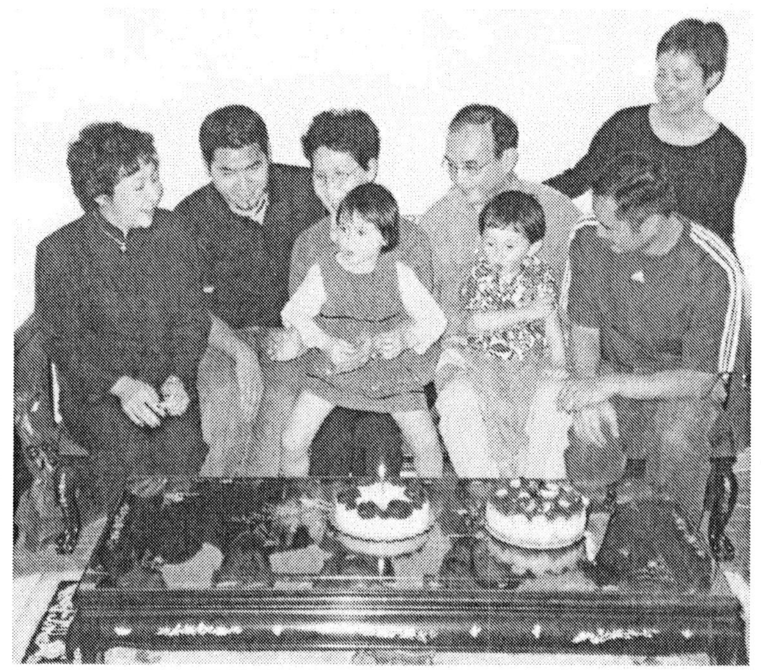

Rosalind Lim (Shaker Heights/Beachwood, Ohio)
Mother of 4 children:
Jonathan-35; Tracy-34; Peter-26; Elizabeth-24

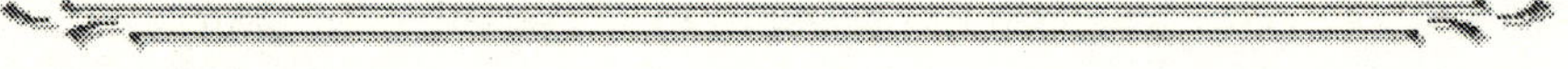

Rosalind Lim, *mother of 4 children - 2 boys and 2 girls (35, 34, 26, 24)*

(Shaker Heights/Beachwood, OH) Age: 58

Southeast Asian - Chinese

> "I was twenty-two when I had my first child. As a new mother, I was not taught by my mother how to breastfeed. Mothers were ashamed to share personal things with their children. However, my oldest daughter did breastfeed her daughter who is now three years old. I told her how important it is to breastfeed. Especially, right after delivery a mother should breastfeed. God created it that way. He created the first milk, which is called the colostrums. Human milk is for humans, cow's milk is for cows, cats' milk is for cats, and dog's milk is for dogs.
>
> Presently, I am a registered nurse. I did breastfeed three of my children for three months. My milk dried up because I did not drink milk or enough fluids while

I was breastfeeding. I was highly sensitive to dairy products. I had to substitute formula milk for them. I try to encourage women to breastfeed their baby after delivery. I tell them you have to give your baby a good start.

Mothers need to breastfeed their baby to develop their immune system to fight illnesses. The immune system is like little soldiers in the line of defense so that viruses cannot penetrate easily. This is the only time that a mother's milk is designed to do that.

Breastfeeding is not easy. It hurts the first time. You just have to bear it for a while. You have to be consistent.

Breastfeeding gives a mother closeness and bonding with the child. The child feels secure when you breastfeed. There is a certain taste that the baby can differentiate between the mother's milk and the formula. The baby has to work much harder with the breast. The baby has to use the jaw muscles and it develops the jaw line.

My first two children are eleven months apart from each other. I did not breastfeed my second child, my daughter. Her immune system is not as strong as my other children. She experienced alopecia, which is a loss of hair. After the doctor was unable to find the solution to help her, I prayed and believed God to help her hair grow back. With the grace of God, her hair grew back.

I encourage pregnant mothers to eat right. I ate plenty of fruits and vegetables along with taking my vitamins. Take your vitamins because our soil is depleted of good nutrition."

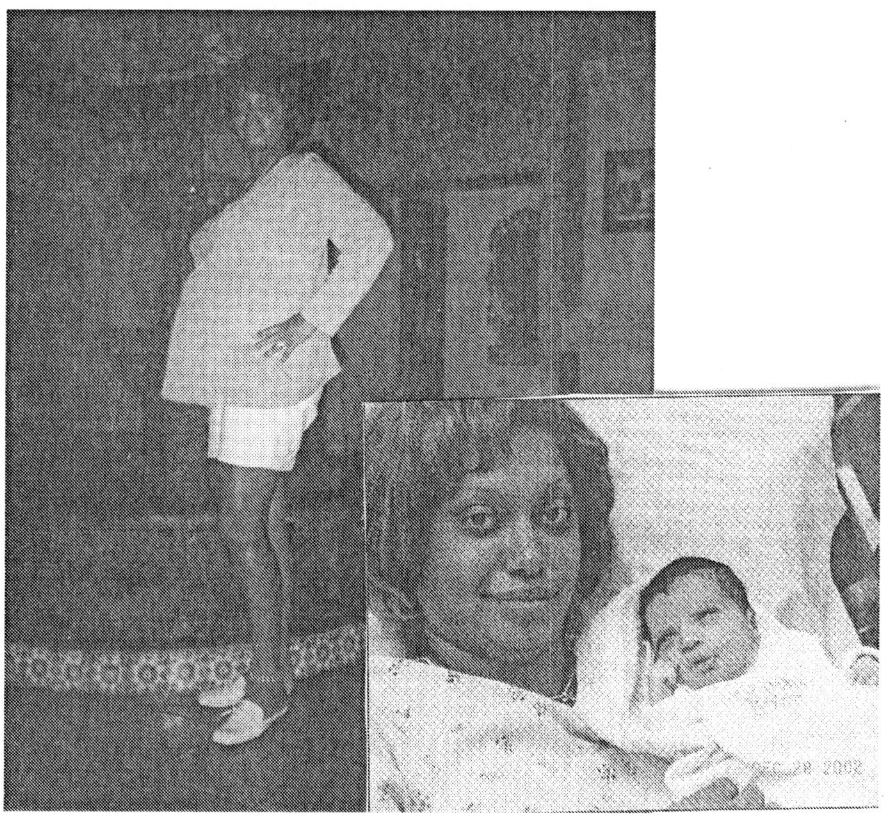

Ramona Lowery (Cleveland, Ohio)
Expecting mother, due date is January 8, 2003
Kayla was born December 28, 2002

Ramona Lowery, *mother of one child, 2 weeks old, (Cleveland, OH) Age: 31*

Person of Color

My decision to breastfed was based on literature I read on the subject. I educated myself early on (before having my baby). Each week I received many e-mails regarding breastfeeding. There were also various magazines with articles on the subject, which I read. The information I read informed me of the fact that breastfed babies had fewer illnesses, let's face it; no one wants a sick child. There was so much medical data that listed the positive benefits, such as a stronger immune system and babies with higher IQ's. It seems as though everything I read was positive.

Even though I was thinking of breastfeeding, I did not make a firm and final decision until after the birth of my child. Now that my baby girl is born, I am breastfeeding. Everything is going fine. I do, however, need support and encouragement as I continue on. I call my family and friends for support and encouragement.

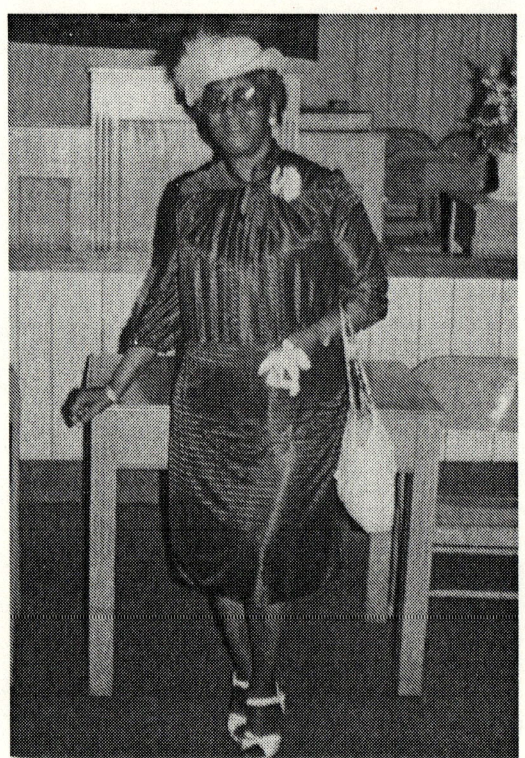

Hattie L. McCreary (Atmore, Alabama)
My grandmother of 9 children
Children not shown here

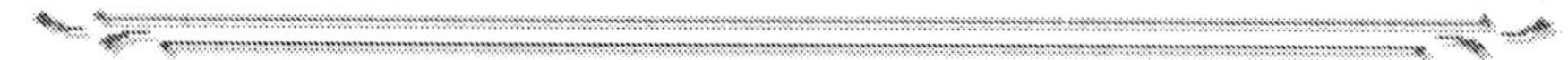

Hattie L. McCreary, ***my grandmother*** *and mother of 9 children, (Atmore, AL) Age: 83*

Person of color

> "If you eat right, babies that are breastfed are healthier than the ones on the bottle. I breastfed all nine of my children and they were smart and healthy. I would do it all over again. It is the best! I encourage all mothers to breastfeed their children."

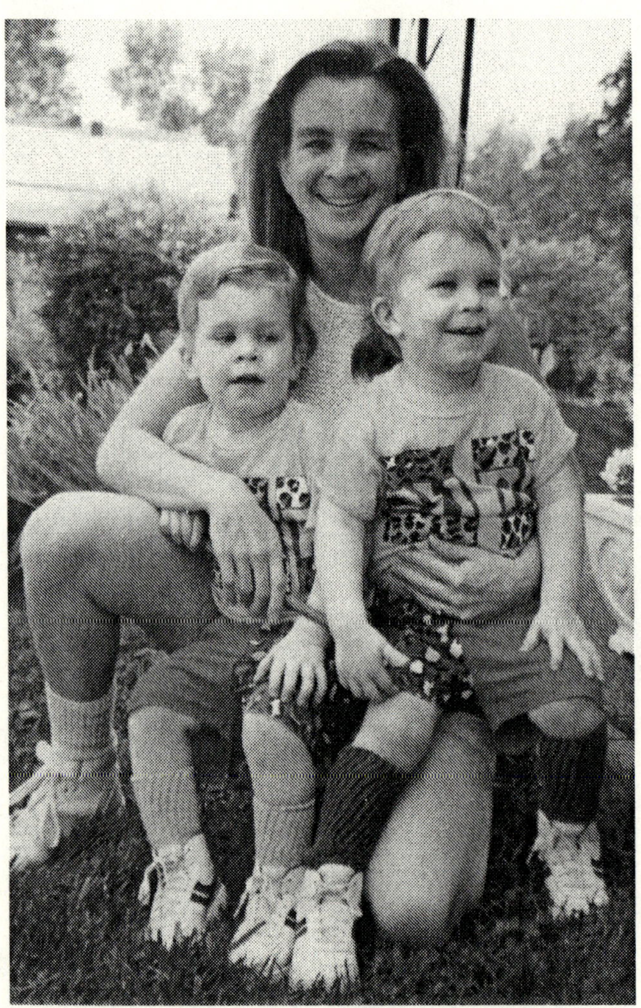

Pastor Pam McKisic (Strongsville, Ohio)
Mother of 4 children:
Twin boys (Joshua and Aaron-14
daughters not shown

Pam McKisic, *mother of 4 children: two girls and twin boys -14 (Strongsville, OH) Age: 46*

Caucasian

"I had the privilege of breastfeeding my older daughter which was over twenty years ago. This I found to be a pleasant experience. When I became pregnant with my sons years later, my pediatrician suggested that I breastfeed my boys. I breast fed my twin boys because I knew it was healthier for them. They were very healthy: no ear infections or diseases, etc. I breast fed because the cost of formula was more expensive and for the closeness and the bonding. Breastfeeding helped me lose the weight I had gained while I was pregnant. I ate healthier during that time. I knew that my milk was giving them more of the nutrients they needed. I breastfed and bottle-fed the twins. I did not have enough milk for them at the same time. I would breastfeed one and bottle-feed the other baby, and then I would switch them for the next feeding. I had the support of my husband and he was in agreement with me breastfeeding the twins. He would also get up at night to help me feed the boys by bringing them to me.

I would encourage any mother to breastfeed their baby. I believe that breastfeeding is how God intended it to be. I enjoyed breastfeeding my twin boys. There was a special bond with them and I really enjoyed holding them close and watching them nurse."

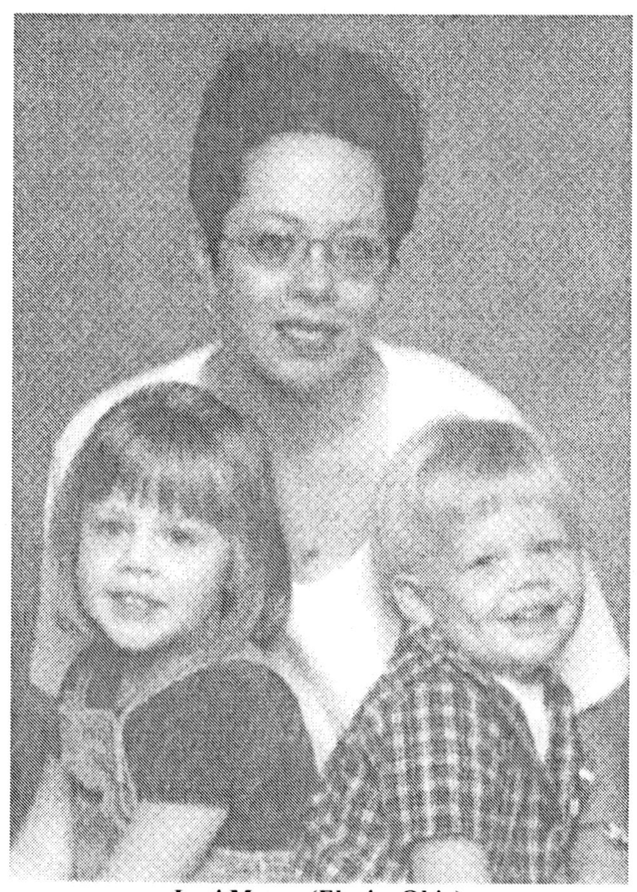

Lori Moore (Elyria, Ohio)
Mother of a girl and boy:
Gabrielle J.-5; Levi F.-3

Lori Moore, *mother of 2 children - boy -3 and girl - 5 (Elyria, OH)*

Age: 32

Caucasian

I breast fed both my daughter, Gabbi and my son, Levi. I did so for eight to ten months each. There is so much good that can come out of it – nutrition, immunities, bonding, and indescribable love. I would recommend breastfeeding to any new mother. In my opinion, there is only good that can come from it! I also did a lot of "pumping" so my husband could have his "special" time feeding them and they would still get the great nutrients of the breast milk. When I lost baby Luke - that is one of the things that I missed the most-that special time alone feeding him and bonding.

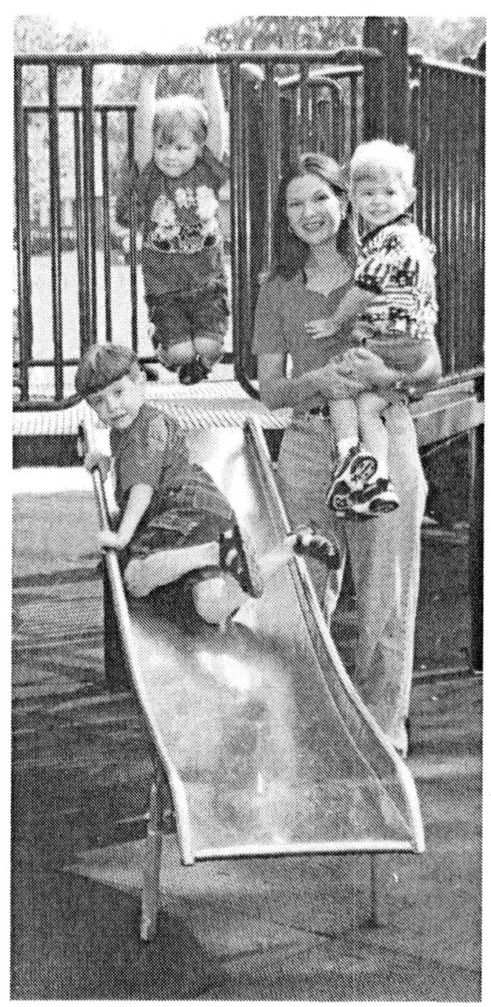

Shelia Moore (Parma, Ohio)
Mother of 3 boys:
Grant-6; Anthony-3; Trey-2

Shelia Moore, *mother of 3 boys – 6, 3, 2 (Parma, OH) Age: 28 Caucasian*

"Breastfeeding my three boys were very rewarding. It is definitely a time I will always cherish. Words cannot come close to describing the special bond that forms and builds between you and your child. It helped me learn to be better in tune to the needs of my baby. God designed breast milk as the *ultimate* nourishment for our babies and it adjusts to fit their needs as they grow. Some keys to successful breastfeeding are to be patient, continue to read and educate yourself, and talk to others who can support you in your decision to nurse. I would encourage any mother to try it!"

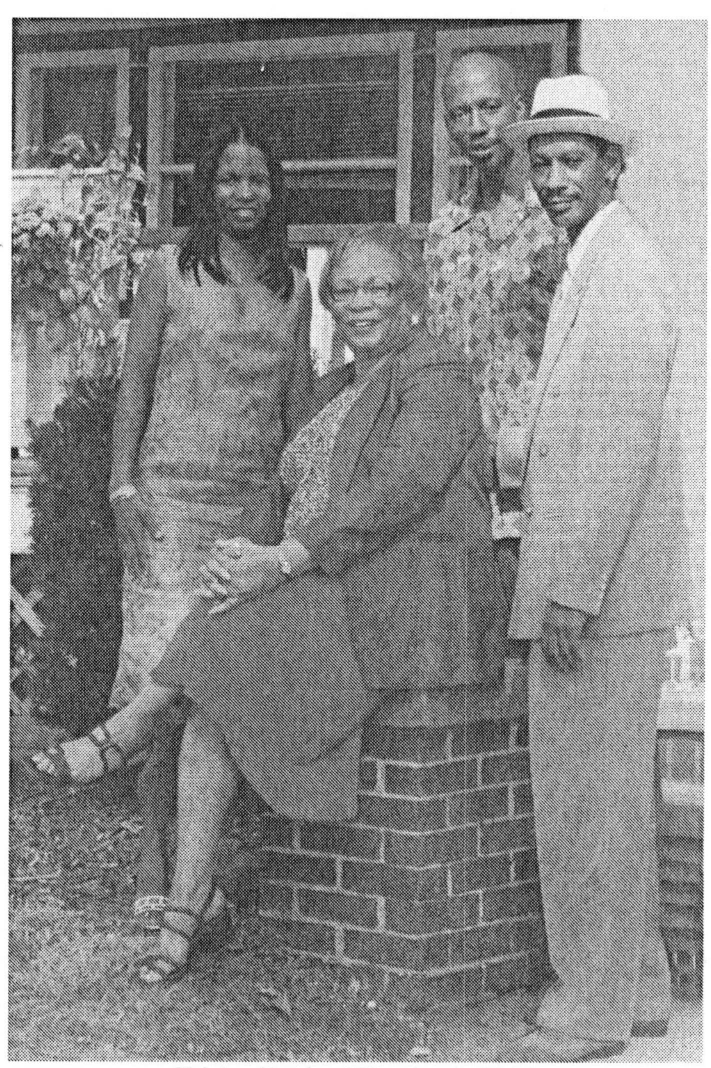

Shirley Napier (Cleveland, Ohio)
Mother of 4 children:
Anthony-46; Timothy-44, Jeffrey-42; Tracye-33
one child not pictured

Shirley Napier, *mother of 4 children - 3 boys and 1 girl - 45, 43, 39, 32*

(Cleveland, OH) Age: 68

Person of Color

"One of my early childhood memories was seeing a mother breastfeed her baby in church. As I remember, there were no disgusting gasps of breath or those "How dare she think she can do that!" kind of looks!" No one appeared to be in a state of shock. Quite frankly I was curious about what was happening.

Our wise Creator designed the most natural, economical, convenient and healthy method of feeding our infants. I observed over the years mans efforts to try and make a better product than the one originated by the Creator of the baby as well as the nourishment needed by him or her.

The times of my nursing was during a period when mothers were falling into society's trap of thinking it was more fulfilling to be working away from home as opposed to being an at home mother raising your children. Sad to say, I was one such mother. Consequently, not every one of my babies received the benefits of being nursed. However, the ones who were fortunate enough to be nursed were not sickly children and bonding with them was much easier. This is an experience that every mother should have if at all possible.

We are living now in a society where there is a lack of priority given to our children. The fast paced lives and the desire for more and more things has lead to an unfulfilled void in the lives of many of our young. I truly believe mothers who will nurture their babies through breastfeeding will have fewer emotional and physical problems from their children later on. This in itself is a positive reason for not falling for what society deems a freedom.

We have allowed society to pervert something beautiful God has given. We have permitted a woman's breast to become and object of sex almost totally. Unfortunately, some men and women alike prefer it this way as opposed to the breast being the God given nourisher for our precious babies both which come from him."

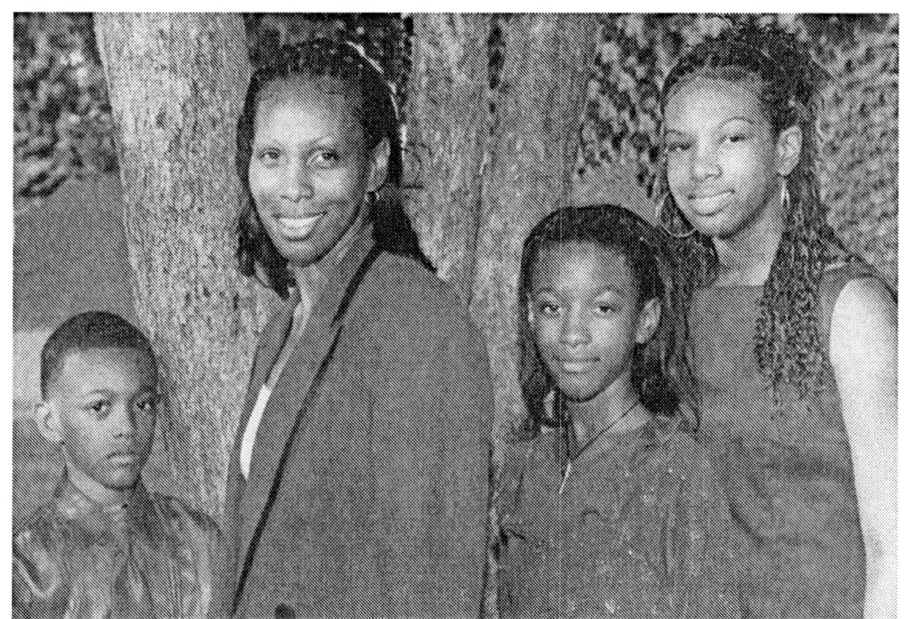

Ronda Naylor (Euclid, Ohio)
Mother of 3 children:
Stacie-15; Tifini-10; Trent-8

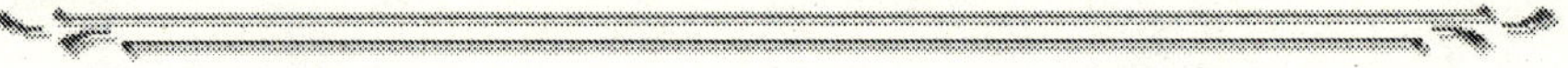

Ronda Naylor, *mother of 3 children - 15, 10, 8 (Euclid, OH) Age: 38*

Person of color

"I am a mother of three children and I am very proud of myself. I began mother hood at the age of 23 years. My oldest is now 15 years old. Nursing my children was the most important thing to me. When I first found out I was pregnant my doctor ask me was I going to breast feed or use formula. After doing a short study on the difference between breast-fed and formula fed babies I was very thoroughly persuaded that breast-feeding was the safest, most secure way to feed my children. Not only did it give me a personal security as far as what I was allowing to go through my innocent little ones bodies, but it gave me something more and that was TIME, personal time with my children. Each one individually had a set time of day that they knew we would be together. That one choice began a relationship for a lifetime."

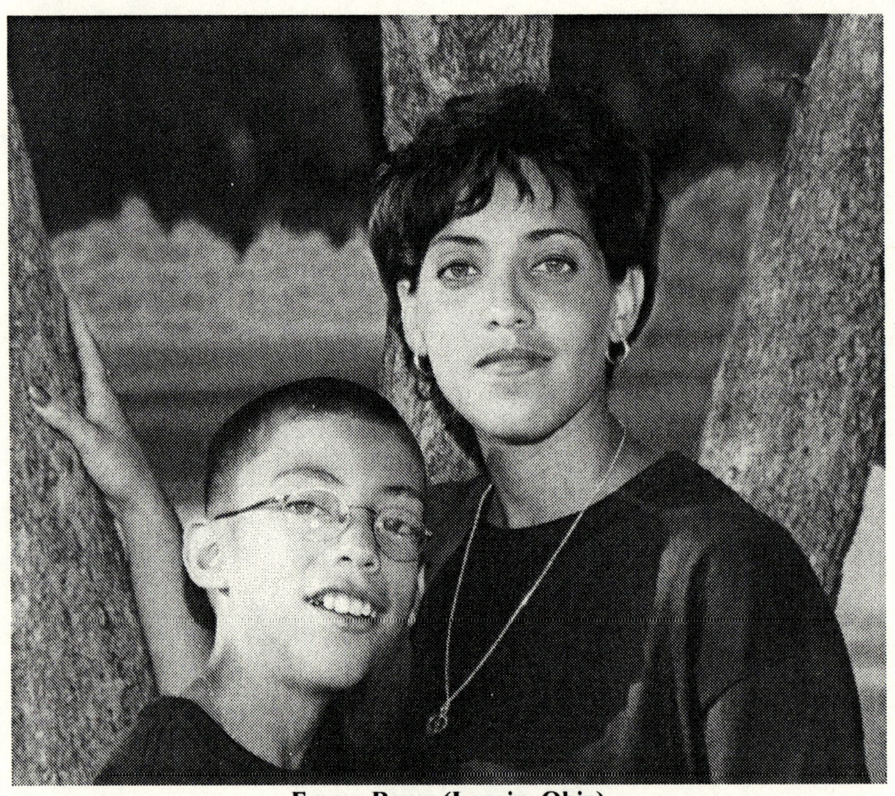

Emmy Reyes (Lorain, Ohio)
Mother of a son and is expecting a child due date December 5, 2002
Tony-8

Emmy Reyes, *mother of 1 child and one in the womb -11 (Lorain, OH) Age: 30*

Hispanic

"I was twenty years old when I had my son Antonio Isaias Reyes. I felt very blessed and excited to be a mom and my goal was to give him all the love; nurturing and caring a mother can give to her baby. I had heard a lot about the benefits of breastfeeding and read some pamphlets. So, I made a decision to do it. Although I had made my decision, I did not have the proper education that a new mom needed to properly breastfeed her baby. I remembered being in the hospital after having a C-section, and the nurse bringing my baby so I could feed him. At that time, I expressed to her that I wanted to breastfeed. She briefly showed me what to do and that was it. I was only able to breastfeed for about two months after which I pumped my breast. This allowed me to give him breast milk for an additional month. I found it hard to do because of my lack of education in this area. I assumed that it was not meant for me.

I am currently expecting my second child. This time I have made sure to read more about it, talk to more women who are breastfeeding, or have successfully done it in the past. I have also become more knowledgeable in how to take care of my body by taking the right supplements and vitamins and eating a good diet. Breastfeeding is a unique experience and it creates a beautiful bond between mom and baby. I believe that every mom should have this wonderful experience and at least try it once."

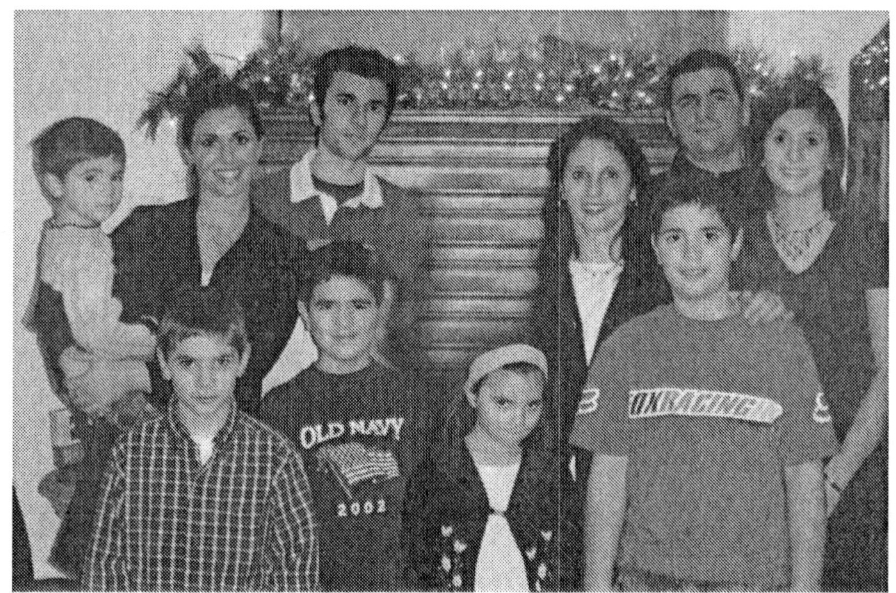

Lynda Romanin (Cleveland Heights, Ohio)
Mother of 9 children:
Angeline-24; Christopher-22; Mark-19; Jacqueline-14;
Jonathan-11; (twin boys) Daniel & Thomas-8;
Christina-6; Brian-4

Lynda Romanin, *mother of 9 children – 24, 22, 19, 14, 11, 8, 8, 6, 4,*

(Cleveland Heights, OH) Age: 47

Greek

"All of these were healthy breastfed babies!" The Lord directed me nurse. I had no mentor to teach me nor had I ever seen anyone breastfed. With Gods leading me, I decided to breastfeed all nine of my children. Their ages range from twenty-four years down to four years of age. I have three girls and six boys with a set of twin boys in the mix. Before my twins were born, I had asked God to make me a woman of faith. The longest period of time I spent nursing any one child was four years. My husband would say at two years, "It is long enough". At three years he would say, "Give it up". I would pray for God to set the time for weaning each baby. He never allowed the weaning to be a traumatic experience for the babies or myself. There was no separation anxiety with any of my children when it was time to wean them. They were all very secure. The shortest period I nursed was for one year. On the advice of my doctor, I stopped nursing because my baby was jaundice. The medical community was not aware at that time that a mother's milk was the absolute best for any child, jaundice or not.

Amid the nine children, I was blessed with twin boys. Not only did all of the children bond to me, the twins bonded with me and with each other. As I fed the two, they would hold hands and this continued for almost three years. None of my children needed to use a pacifier. Consequently, this was not a habit that had to be broken later on.

There were no problems with them drinking after the weaning process. They all took readily to carrot juice and protein drinks in place of my milk. Fresh fruits and vegetables took the place of baby food in a jar. My children never drank cow's milk. We were designed by God to nourish our own children with our own milk. All other animals are fed only their mother's milk. That should really say something to us as human beings.

As I related earlier, I asked God to make me a woman of faith. He did! One of my constant sayings is "Let's see what God will do!" I cannot encourage you enough to pray and ask for His guidance and wisdom when it comes to raising your children. I had no older woman to guide or disciple me. I had to depend on God. Not only was my nursing time, a time to nourish my babies; it was also a quiet time I spent with God. I had to become a woman of faith.

I had only God to trust when I had two miscarriages in a matter of months. I went it God in fasting and prayer after having gone through this trial. When I emerged from this time with God, I found that I was pregnant again. This happened all within a matter of weeks. I sensed the Lord say that He would give those two babies back to me. I desired to have a natural birth at home and this prayer was partially answered when God sent into my life an OBGYN nurse and her friend. They became my midwives and were of immeasurable help and support when the twins were born.

At the insistence of my husband, I agreed to an ultrasound even though my trust was in the Lord that all was well. I was considered high risk after a brief ultrasound was taken and two babies were discovered on the scene. The Lord touched my husband's heart at that point to allow me to have the babies at home. Trusting God, my babies were born two hours apart, weighing in at eight and one half pounds each. For twelve long hours after the births, the placenta would not pass. After calling people to pray for me, my husband who has been such a support in all of my childbirths saved the day, "With Gods help, of course!" Tired and worn from this ordeal, I fainted. He proceeded to pick me up and in the process he stepped on the umbilical cord and released that which I had held those twelve long hours. Imagine this, I was able to have one child latch on and feed right away. However, the other twin had his first meal "dining out". Another nursing mom had to give him his first nourishment (this is like a wet-nurse). I had no other problem feeding him from that time until he was weaned.

May I say you need those around you who are willing and able to give you the support you need. A little encouragement never hurts. Some benefits of nursing include its quickness and the night sessions are not difficult to endure. You are always in a state of readiness. Believe it or not, I have walked to the store nursing. I have nursed in the store, while I shopped, as well as in church. I have always been covered and discreet when I was feeding my babies. People were never aware of what I was doing. They just thought the babies were asleep under the blanket. Slings come highly recommended because they allow for privacy as well as intimacy when you are nursing.

Please do not neglect your body. Take time for yourself. This is an absolute must. I had no problems with sickness or breast infections. The weight that I gained, I lost quickly. Eating healthy and taking your vitamins is a must. There are many herbal teas such as a raspberry leaf tea and blessed thistle that I drank when nursing. These help increase the supply of the milk to the breast. My milk was in full demand, for you see at times the next baby was on the way while I was still nursing. Sometimes there were two instead of one nursing at the same time. God is not in short supply of anything.

Pray and ask Him to guide you: "Let's see what God will do."

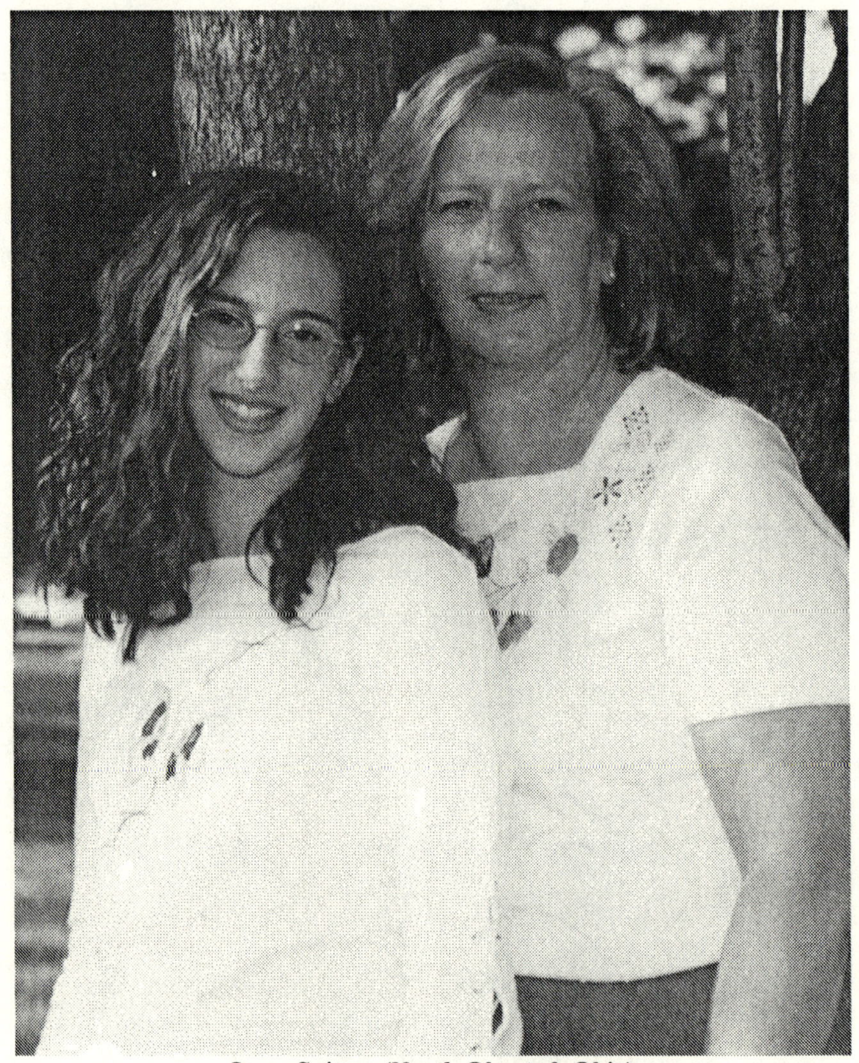

Joyce Spitzer (North Olmsted, Ohio)
Mother of 3 children:
Veronica-33; Richard-26; April-13
Two children not pictured

Joyce Spitzer, *mother of 3 children - 33, 26, 13, (North Olmsted, OH) Age: 54*

Messianic/Jew

"I nursed two of my three children. Our first child had a lot of asthma and allergy problems. The next two I nursed; their health was dramatically different. My second child had only minor asthma and allergy problems compared to my first child. Our third child had no asthma problems at all. Nursing my children was very beneficial to their health. There are a lot of allergies and asthma in the family.

By the time I had my third child, I had learned a lot about supplements and how I could be healthier and have healthier children."

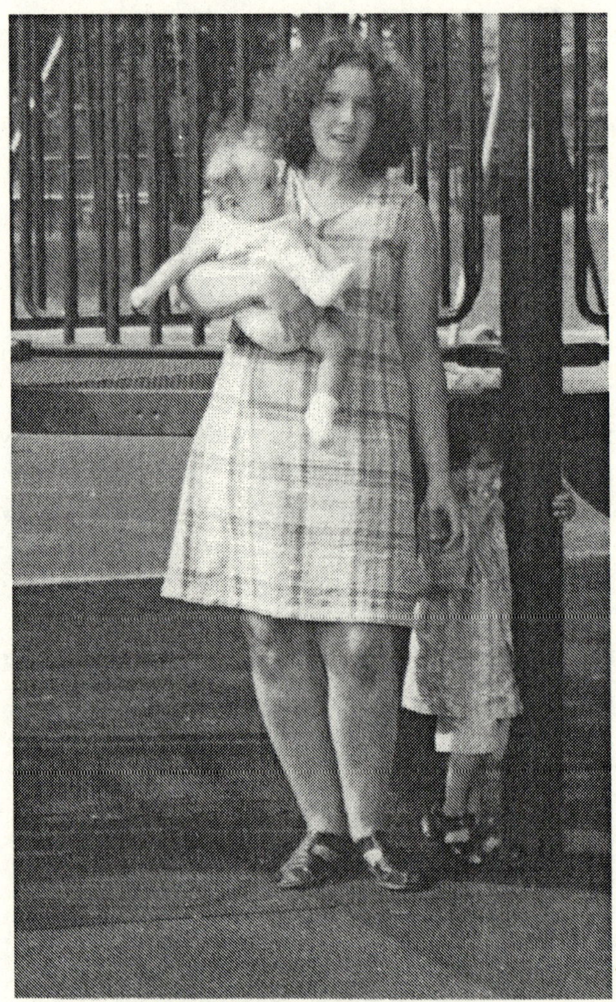

Heather Wilcox (Cleveland, Ohio)
Mother of a boy and girl:
Tyler Matthew-2 ½; Halle-6 months

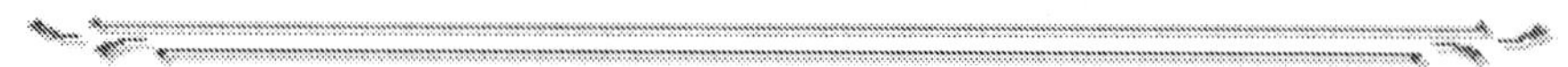

Heather Wilcox, *mother of a son & a daughter – 2 ½, 4 months (Cleveland, OH) Age: 26*

Hispanic

"Breastfeeding your baby is one of the most beneficial, loving, and natural experiences you can ever have. Tyler was breastfed until he was four months old. Now, at age two and one half, he is far more intelligent than most children his age. I credit a lot of this to breastfeeding. To this day, my son and I share a special bond together because of breastfeeding."

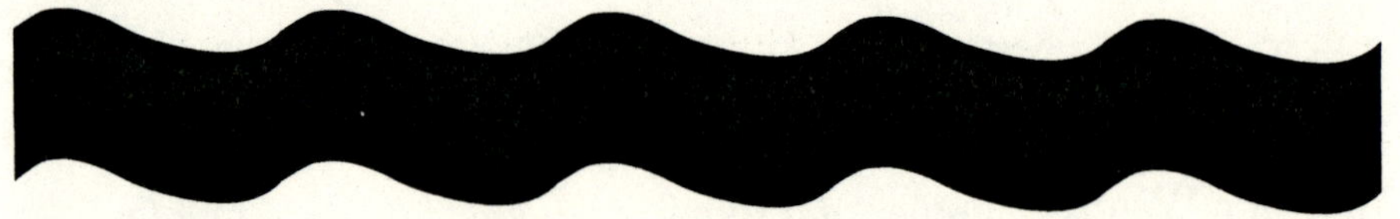

CHAPTER EIGHT

WHY NOT BREASTFEED?

Ninety- nine percent of mothers who want to nurse are physically able to breastfeed their baby. They just do not know it! For many mothers, it requires a lot of time and patience to breastfeed. However, many women today consider breastfeeding because it is a natural process for feeding their children and it brings the child closer to the mother.[44]

There could be several reasons why you may not want to nurse your baby. You may feel it will hamper your lifestyle and take away the freedom and control that you now may enjoy. Those things could be distractions from the devil to keep your mind in darkness. You must change your mind and attitude in order for God to operate in

[44] Healthy Expectations, p. 215

your life as a nursing mother. This is a small sacrifice to make in your life. The majority of my research sources encourage a mother to eat healthy while the baby is in the womb as well as when they are breastfeeding. This allows the mother to give her baby the best from the very beginning.

I challenge you to become the Virtuous Woman that is spoken of in the Book of Proverbs. The following verses of scripture emphasize the importance of the mother in the home. Ask the Lord to show you how to apply these scriptures in your life today!

(Proverbs 31: 10-31 KJV) says:

Who can find a virtuous woman? For her price is far above rubies. The heart of her husband doth safely trust in her, so that he shall have no need of spoil. She will do him good and not evil all the days of her life. She seeketh wool, and flax, and worketh willingly with her hands. She is like the merchants ships; she bringeth her food from afar. She riseth also while it is yet night, and giveth meat to her household and a portion to her maidens. She considereth a field, and buyeth it: with the fruit of her hands she planteth a vineyard. She girdeth her loins with strength, and strengtheneth her arms. She perceiveth that her merchandise is good: her candle goeth not out by night. She layeth her hands to the spindle, and her hands hold the distaff. She stretcheth out her hand to the poor; yea, she reacheth forth her hands to the needy. She is not afraid of the snow for her household: for all her household are clothed with scarlet. She maketh herself coverings of tapestry; her clothing is silk and purple. Her husband is known in the gates, when he sitteth among the elders of the land. She maketh fine linen, and selleth it; and delivereth girdles unto the merchant. Strength and honor are her clothing; and she shall rejoice in the time to come. She openeth her mouth with wisdom; and in her tongue is the law of kindness. She looketh well to the ways of her household, and eateth not the bread of idleness. Her children arise up, and call her blessed;

her husband also, and he praiseth her. Many daughters have done virtuously, but thou excellest them all. Favor is deceitful, and beauty is vain: but a woman that feareth the Lord, she shall be praised. Give her of the fruit of her hands; and let her own works praise her in the gates.

(Proverbs 14:1 KJV) says:

Every wise woman buildeth her house: but the foolish plucketh it down with her hands.

Build your house by not allowing perverted thinking against nursing your baby to distract you from God's plan and purpose for your life and your child's life.

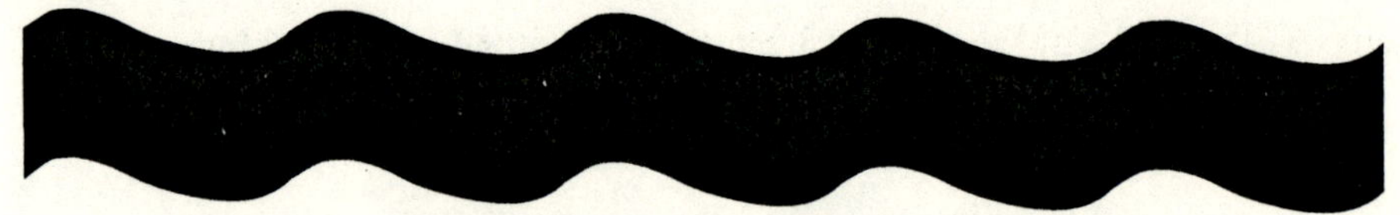

CHAPTER NINE

THE PROS AND CONS OF BREASTFEEDING

By now you can see that I strongly believe in the benefits of breast milk for my babies. What God has designed has enabled me to give my son and daughter the very best nutrition. For me, breastfeeding is a biological function of my womanhood. I have sincerely benefited from using this function of my body. I was created to nurture life and given breasts to nourish that life, which are my children. I do not want to be disobedient to what The word of God says by turning away from His instruction when it comes to breastfeeding. I felt that if I blatantly refused to nurse my baby after praying and asking God to give me the strength to do this and informing myself regarding breastfeeding I would go against God's plan for me as a mother/woman.

To those women who are physically unable to produce milk for their babies and have a desire to give them breast milk; there are some alternatives for these mothers such as a Human Milk Bank that is supplied by mothers who donate their excess breast milk. The mothers' milk that is sent to the banks is tested for safety. Human Milk Banking is a service, which collects, screens, processes, and dispenses by prescription human milk donated by nursing mothers who are not biologically related to the recipient infant. [45]

Some hospitals can attach small syringe like tubes to the mothers' breast with milk flowing through the tubes so that your baby can have the skin-to-skin closeness. This can be done until the mothers' milk begins to flow. The pulling on the nipple helps stimulate the milk ducts so that milk can come down. Adoptive mothers can benefit from these options if they are interested in breast milk for their baby. These alternatives may also apply to women who have had mastectomies or who are on medication that would be detrimental to the heath of the baby. If you are interested in using one of these options, please talk to your doctor regarding what is available. Many doctors are not aware that human milk banks exist in America. Being informed about breastfeeding your baby could be a tremendous plus.

---

[45] Human Milk Banks, www.cdc.gov, p. 1-6

Therefore, here are some things you may consider in making your decision to breastfeed your infant:

When a mother is nursing her baby, the hormone prolactin, is operating. This is a very strong "love hormone" which bonds the mother to her baby. Animal studies regarding this hormone are most interesting. When it is injected into a rooster, it will make the rooster become clucky and mother the chickens! How about that? A female animal that is nursing her young in the wild will fight to the death any intruder upon her young, whereas after weaning, she does not show this protection. The mother who is nursing her baby is bound to her baby. She finds it hard to leave her baby with a baby-sitter. This is God's powerful plan. He does not intend for mothers to leave their babies after a few months to pursue their career. Mothers already have a more important career. Breastfeeding ties them to each another.[46] There is another hormone, oxytocin, which is released by the pituitary gland. This is the hormone that stimulates the mother's letdown or milk-ejection reflex (the tingly sensation you feel when the milk lets down). This is a wonderful hormone that has a calming affect upon

---

[46] www.aboverubies.com, Breastfeeding God's Way

the mother. Every time the milk lets down, the mother experiences a feeling of relaxation and calm and sometimes sleepiness comes over her. God is good because of all the information He has allowed the medical profession to discover which benefit the nursing mother. When we do things God's way, we get His benefits. He knows that mothers need this calming hormone and He has graciously provided it for you and me![47]

THINGS TO CONSIDER FOR BREASTFEEDING OR BOTTLE FEEDING:

BOTTLE FEEDING Pros:

1. It allows the father to share the feeding responsibilities and the benefits of bonding more easily.
2. Today's formulas are closely approximated to the nutritional composition of breast milk, although, they cannot provide all the benefits of your custom-made milk.

[47] www.aboverubies.com, Breastfeeding God's Way

3. It does not tie the mother down. You are able to work outside the home, shop, go out in the evening, or even sleep through the night because someone else can feed the baby.
4. It does not interfere with a couples' sex life unless the baby wakes up for a feeding at the wrong time.[48]
5. It does not dictate your diet or alter your style of eating. You can eat all the garlic, spicy foods, and cabbage etc. that you desire.
6. You do not have to drink any milk or restrict your intake of other beverages.
7. May be preferable for a woman who is hesitant having such intimate contact with her infant.
8. Mothers may feel uncomfortable about the possibility of nursing in public.
9. A mother who feels she is too high-strung or impatient to breastfeed.[49]

[48] Healthy Expectation, p. 214-215
[49] What To Expect When You're Expecting, p. 253

10. Some professionals seem to think formula is a superior form of nutrition for babies.[50]
11. Some professionals seem to think babies who are fed formulas appear to be just as healthy as breastfed babies.[51]

BOTTLE FEEDING Cons:

1. The inconvenience of daily bottle preparation. Clean and sterilize the bottles.
2. The cost of bottles and nipples and other tools needed for preparation.
3. The baby has to wait to be fed.
4. Bottles must be heated to the right temperature.
5. Fear of falling asleep.
6. Having to watch the number of ounces the baby takes.
7. Nipple holes may be too small or too large.
8. Fear of baby sucking in uncomfortable amounts of air.

---

[50] A Doctor Discusses Nutrition During Pregnancy & Breast Feeding, p. 81

[51] A Doctor Discusses Nutrition During Pregnancy & Breast Feeding, p. 81

9. The necessity of burping each time they feed.
10. Frustration and anxiety in choosing a satisfactory formula.
11. You must buy the formula which is expensive.[52]
12. Someone expends time to purchase formula.
13. Cost is well over $1000 per year (not including the extra expenses to the doctor's office when you treat the formula fed baby who is more prone to sickness).[53] There have been recalls on formulas.
14. The return of menstrual cycle is not delayed.
15. Formula based on cow's milk may irritate the gut, causing a loss of blood and increasing the risk of anemia.
16. Babies can become sensitized (and allergic) to cow's milk or soymilk.
17. Allergies to latex (bottle nipples and pacifiers are made of latex).[54]
18. The fats most often used in formula are cottonseed oil, beef tallow, and coconut oil.[55]

---

[52] A Doctor Discusses Nutrition During Pregnancy & Breast Feeding, p. 104-108
[53] Compassionate Souls, p. 29
[54] Compassionate Soul, p. 34
[55] Compassionate Souls, p. 27

19. You can overfeed on formula.

BREASTFEEDING Pros:

1. Contains essential fatty acids not found in formula.
2. Essential fatty acids are necessary for development of the brain and retina.
3. Breast milk contains an extremely absorbable form of iron.[56]
4. Breast milk is a food and a medicine.
5. Allows baby to nurse when desired.
6. It is not possible to overfeed.
7. Baby can relax.
8. Mother can relax.
9. The baby learns to honor their own body signals because the water content, fat, and other nutritional parameters of breast milk fluctuate to meet the baby's changing needs (thirst, hunger, comfort).[57]

---

[56] Compassionate Souls, p. 33
[57] Compassionate Souls, p. 36

BREASTFEEDING Cons:

1. If you are using certain medications that would be harmful to the baby.
2. Eating certain types of foods that may affect the baby.
3. Not being able to feed in a moving automobile.

According to the United Nations Children's Fund (UNICEF), one and one half million babies die each year because they are not breastfed.[58]

If you chose to breastfeed your baby, you can and will be able to continue with loving support from your husband, family, or close friends. They are the ones who can and will encourage you. **You can do it!** Start today getting your milk-manufacturing machine in proper working order. Do not forget to nourish your body with plenty of fresh fruits and vegetables. Drink plenty of water (H_20), the heavenly drink given from the Creator.

You will appreciate the benefits of what God has provided for a nursing mother once you educate yourself. Put it into practice!

---

[58] Compassionate Souls, p. 28

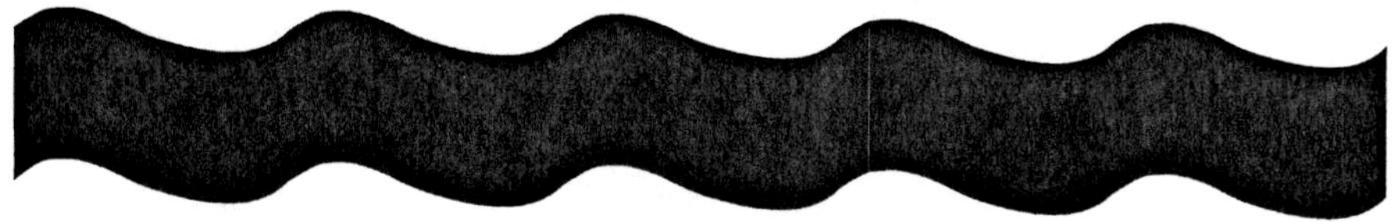

CHAPTER TEN

MY SECOND CHILD

There is definite a difference between the breastfeeding and health of my second child as opposed to my first child. My second child is a girl who is beautiful and a precious jewel from the Lord. She arrived at a moment that my husband and I deemed to be a very low point in our life!

Because our financial status had decreased, I did not eat and take my necessary vitamins the way I did with my son. My diet was not as healthy nor was my water consumption as with my son. With my daughter, I ate whatever I could to keep myself from being hungry. I took the most important vitamin, which was the multivitamin.

During this time in my life, it was extremely difficult physically and emotionally. Judging between the two pregnancies, I ate the things I needed as well as the ones I craved with my son. The state of our finances determined my ability to satisfy my cravings with my daughter. I basically ate whatever was available to me at that time.

I was extremely healthy with my son. I was always eating. Day and night, I ate. It seemed as though I could not get enough food. I consumed a considerable amount of food with my daughter. But, it was not the same. My stomach would growl continually. I never seemed to be able to satisfy my hunger. I can laugh about it now, but it was far from being funny then. There were times when my husband had to make me a sandwich in the middle of the night because I was so hungry.

I weighed one hundred and ten pounds before I became pregnant, so I could afford to gain some weight. However, I did not gain a lot of weight with my baby girl. I gained twenty-eight pounds with my daughter and forty-two pounds with my son. That was a considerable amount of pounds for my small frame. Doctors recommend that you only gain up to thirty pounds. My belief is that the amounts I ate contributed to the difference between their sizes, health, and how they nursed.

My daughter was born very tiny and had bags underneath her eyes. She was born at five pounds, thirteen ounces versus my son, being born at one ounce shy of eight pounds. Also, a heart specialist diagnosed her as having a hole in her heart that was larger than normal. My husband and I are trusting God to close it before she is one-year- old.

I truly believe that this was because of my eating habits and the fact that I was stressed due to our financial pressures. Not having the money to purchase many things I needed when I was pregnant made a big difference with our health. My husband was facing difficult challenges on the new job he had recently taken and this did not help my stress level. He was not getting the salary that he received at his previous job, which made a huge difference in our living situation.

Worrying and stressing over all these things, I experienced extreme lower back pain and severe headaches most the time. Before my daughter was born, it became necessary for me to see a massage therapist for my back once a week. The therapist was feeling mostly baby and very little amniotic fluid in my womb as she massaged me. I was all baby! I could feel the baby resting on my back and tailbone. I considered that to be a miracle, to carry my baby with such a small amount of fluid!

My daughter did not have a problem breastfeeding when the nurse brought her to me for her first feeding. She latched on right away just as her brother was able to do. By the way, when she came out of the womb, she was smacking her lips. She must have been very hungry. However, she did not eat as much as my son did on his first try. My son would empty both breast within ten minutes. She still does not eat very much at one time. She is more of a snacker. She eats when she is ready to eat! Only if she is really hungry, will she drain one breast and save the other for later.

Having a glass or a bottle of water to drink while you are nursing helps dispel dry mouth and possible headaches. These can cause your nursing experience to be less than pleasant

You must be mindful of the foods you eat that give any indication that your baby is having some sort of reaction. I discovered that my eating tuna fish and pineapples for two or three week's straight did possibly cause a reaction in her skin. This also became true when I ingested a whole delicious mango. This same day I ate more fish, mind you, and I was already eating a great deal of tuna sandwiches.

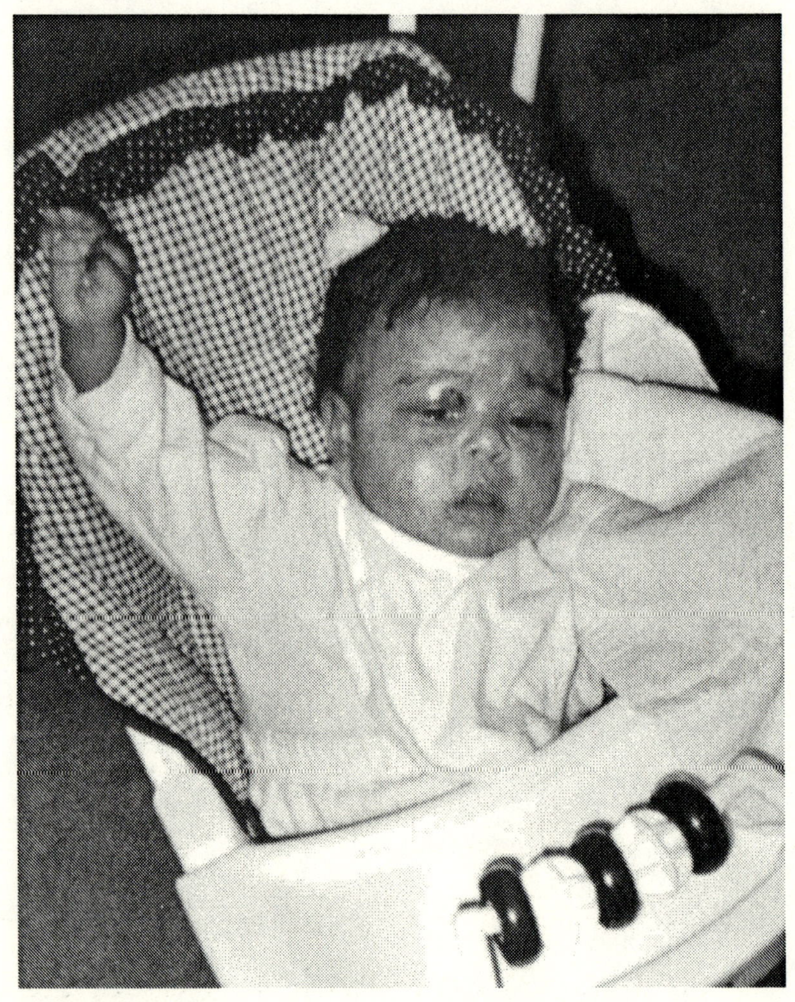

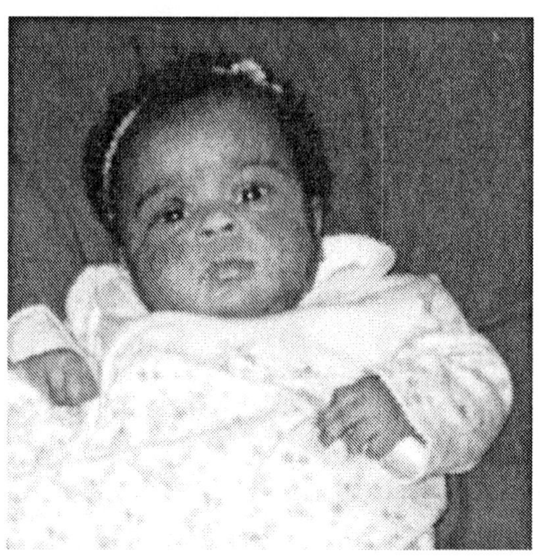

That evening I began to notice my daughter breaking out in little bumps on her face. I thought it was just a heat rash, or the changes that newborns go through with their skin. I continued to bathe her daily; using the same brand of baby washes and baby oil on her skin. Gradually I started seeing more bumps developing and white patches on her face. So, I tried coco butter, to see if that would help clear up the rash. It did not. Then, it began to get worse. I bathed her body with a new baby wash and it seemed to get better. So, I thought everything was okay with her skin.

Again I began to notice that my daughters face was looking even worse than before. Her face had the appearance of having been burned. Her skin became very tender, scaly, red, and wet. You could see the nerves in her face because the skin had begun to peel away. This same burned look, invaded her buttock area as well as her scalp. There were sores on her eyes that kept bleeding. If you touched them in the wrong way, the blood would pour out of them. Everywhere you could imagine (chest, shoulders, ears, toes, neck); she was breaking out. All of these areas were affected. She was in a miserable state at this point and I was just as miserable having to look at her, unable to help. It was hard for her to smile, nurse, or cry. I would have to cleanse her face frequently to try and soothe her skin. This would work for a while and then we would have to start the cleansing process all over again. I tried everything that I thought would clear up her condition to no avail. My husband and I prayed for her everyday, believing that the Lord would heal her body and give us wisdom about what to do. When I took her to the pediatrician, she could not examine her at that time. Her nurse advised me to try a product called Aquafor. I did and it kept her face from chapping or cracking, but it did not clear her skin. I ended up taking her to the emergency room where they could only say that it was some type of dermatitis, for which they prescribed a bacteria crème. They suggested that I take her to a pediatrician if it did not heal. I took her to the pediatrician for a follow-up visit. The pediatrician saw her and she was unable to give a clear diagnosis. A blood sample and swab sample were taken from her face for the lab to determine if there was an infection. Her toe was badly infected and her face proved to be infected also. The pediatrician wanted a dermatologist to see her, but at that time he was not available. So, she prescribed for her penicillin and two types of creams. My daughter's skin was still not clear after having used the medication except for a few places on her toe and under her chin. The doctor then suggested I see another dermatologist because he did not know what to do and he had never seen anything like this before.

On the advice of my hair stylist, I took her to a dermatologist that he knew and came highly recommended. When this doctor saw her, right away, he knew what the problem was and wanted to have her blood tested. It appeared to him that she had a zinc deficiency and in addition, there was a yeast infection from the penicillin that had been prescribed previously. The penicillin had caused the thrush in her mouth and on her tongue. The doctor had her zinc count tested which confirmed the diagnosis he had already given. Her zinc level was at sixteen and the normal count for an infant is seventy. He then prescribed her a liquid zinc mineral, bacteria cream for her eyes, and cortisone crème for her skin. When I took her back for her follow-up visit, her zinc level was up to where it was suppose to be and her face was clearing up quickly. The doctor said she looked so much better and appeared happier. My baby was eating more, laughing and smiling again.

Several people believed God with us that she was already healed. Halleluiah, the Lord answered all of our prayers.

I share this testimony with you to let you know that as mothers we need to eat a healthy diet, and study about breastfeeding. I believed that the mango may have triggered something in her body along with too much tuna fish and pineapples.

Eat healthy, eat right, and take your vitamins while you are pregnant and nursing your infant. Bless the Lord, she has no scars from this ordeal and her clear skin complexion has returned. The rash had taken her hair out in the spots, now her hair is growing back beautifully. She is beautiful and I thank the Lord every day when I look at her face and into her eyes. I make sure that I eat the right foods that I feel will not cause an allergic reaction in her body. If you know that your child has an allergy or could be allergic to certain foods, do not eat them **period!** Remember everything you eat goes into your infant. Pray about what you should eat for yourself and your baby. This is a vital opportunity for you to strengthen his or her immune system. I do not want any mother to experience what I have gone through with my baby girl.

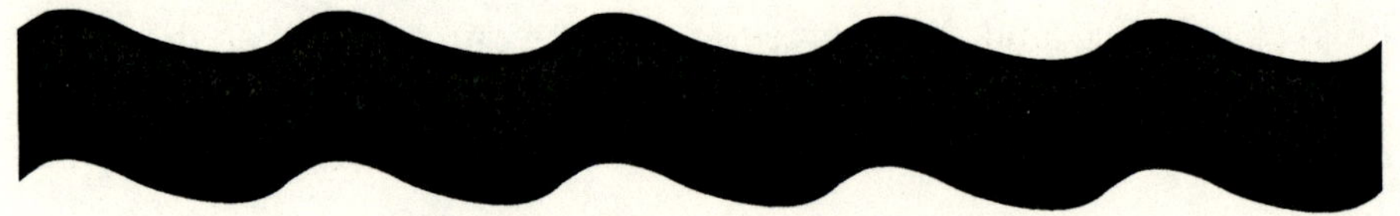

CHAPTER ELEVEN

STAY-AT-HOME MOTHER

(Titus 2:5 KJV) says: To be discreet, chaste, keepers at home, good, obedient to their own husbands, that the word of God be not blasphemed.

My children are a gift to my husband and I from the Lord. Therefore, my gift of love back to God is to breastfeed! God's plan is for mothers to be nurturers in the home and in society. Once my baby was born, I began nurturing my baby at my breast. By being a stay at home mother, I am able to nurture my children in the things of the Lord. I am able to breastfeed on demand if need be because my daughter requires me to feed her promptly. Unlike my son, she does not nurse every three hours. As I stated before she is a snacker.

Working a career job would not allow me to breastfeed on demand. Pumping would not work for her because of the attention she needs and the comforting that it takes for her personality.

Being at home allows me to teach my children how to talk, read, write, cook, and clean. This is all part of home schooling. They learn moral values as I teach them the Bible. As a result of this teaching, they are learning how to live a God fearing life. A strong sense of family, as well as their ability to socialize with others in a respectful way is being instilled in them. No career can take the place of these valuable results. Society has told many mothers it is okay to sacrifice the wellbeing of our children. We have placed them on the altar to be burned instead of our furthered education and careers. They are on the altar in place of the long hours of working harder than everyone else at the office. This is so we can move up the corporate ladder. Mothers are also told they should never depend on a man to take care of them. In all actuality, our total dependence should be on God. Consequently, we sing "God bless the child who has his own". Our children cry from the altar of sacrifice for their own parents and not a hired babysitter. This was the ultimate insult to God's Word when people were advising me to go back to work because of my engineering degree and let my husband stay home and raise the children. That is totally against what God's Word instructs. God gave man a job before he gave him a wife. Will we do it God's way or will we listen to a rebellious society? This is what our generation is telling us in order to be a strong woman. However, God says differently in the scriptures. His Word tells us to be a virtuous woman, that …a wise woman builds her house, and should be keepers at home.

In today's culture, most mothers are not encouraged to stay at home. It is sometimes said, "You cannot survive on one income!" "Thc two of you must work!" You have so many voices speaking so many negative things that it makes you feel as if what you are doing is wrong.

Listen to a story of a mother (Lori Moore) who was in the workforce and after the unfortunate experience of induced labor, birthed a stillborn son.

"God is in control and He will never give me more than what I could handle. Thankfully I decided to hold my breathless son, it was heart breaking and reassuring at the same time. I was angry that my son was taken from me but happy knowing that he was in Heaven, in no pain, being rocked by Jesus!"

"On the way home from the hospital the next day, I knew in my heart that I was not to go back to work. In that short time Baby Luke taught me that it was imperative that I spend all the time I could with my other two children, I had already lost so much time being away from them working! At this point, I truly understood the precious gifts that God intended children to be. God was continuing to expand my territory."

"Now over a year later, I am still at home with Gabbi and Levi. We are having fun, playing, home schooling and just spending time together. I feel it is an awesome privilege to be told by my 3-year-old son that he "needs" me and I can say, "Mommy is right here, honey." God is so good! During bedtime prayer we often thank God that Baby Luke did not have to suffer, that he is in Heaven. "Thank You Jesus!"

I am not materialistic, and I have to do without some things. I am not a pampered mother who sits on my derriere, and devour sweets all day. I am a mother who has completely rearranged her life in order to live on one income. My husband does not make a large amount of money so that it would be convenient for me to stay at home. This was a choice we made because of our faith in my God. I do work!; All day! I just do not get paid for it with dollars. I am rewarded by being obedient to the Lord. I want my children to rise up and call me blessed as it says in Proverbs 31:28. Furthermore, I know I am called to be a stay at home mother. We are anointed to be mothers! I take the responsibility gladly and humbly with my whole heart. It is simple to do if mothers will yield their heart to the Lord by praying and spending time in his Word. I will continue always to do this because I am the handmaid of the Lord.

(Luke 1:38 KJV) says:

> *"Behold the handmaid of the Lord; be it unto me according to thy word"*

This is a good life. I would not trade it for anything. However, remember to take time out for yourself! Whether you are just sitting in the tub relaxing or taking a walk, it gives you time to be alone. Even try napping with your children. This can be very refreshing. Being a mother makes my life very meaningful. I know that motherhood is truly a calling from our awesome Creator. God gives me the strength to continue from day to day.

After I had my first child, my intention was to go back to work and place my child in day care. I have an Electrical Engineer Degree and I was working at General Electric Company at the time and my thought was continuing to work and climb the corporate ladder. You may be saying I may never be able to work again outside the home! You may have gifts talents, and skills that you can use to bring finances into your home by doing a home-based business part-time. However, God spoke to my heart after I had my son. I had peace to come home by faith knowing that the Lord will provide for us if I would be obedient to what he had told me to do. My husband was in agreement with the decision I made to stay at home. I truly thought this was the ultimate sacrifice by relinquishing my financial independence to the Lord and my husband. This was tough! I am glad I decided to stay at home. It has been such a blessing to me to see my children grow in the things of God.

I knew that I would be persecuted for my decision in every possible way, with people's words, my thoughts, and the other outside voices that come to distract me. Sometimes it is very difficult because of the cares of the world that we allow to worry us. I know that it takes money for most things in life. But, I have to trust God no matter what, because He promised that He would provide all of my needs according to His riches in glory by Christ Jesus. He knows all of my needs even when it seems as though I cannot make it or that I am about to lose everything I have. Jesus is the answer! I would rather have the Lord more than anything else. God told me that if I put the word of God in my son first, everything else would come, such as schooling, sports, etc. So this is what I am trying to do daily.

My being at home enables me to monitor what my children watch and hear. I can control what they are exposed to. I do not relinquish that control by putting them under someone else's care. I know what they are learning and their soul is being nurtured.

Experts say mothers who choose to leave the workforce to rear their children are winning on two fronts: they have less stress, and they have healthier, happier husbands. University of Chicago sociologist Linda Waite, co-director of Alfred P. Sloan Center on Parents, Children and Work, researched five-hundred families nationwide and concluded: "In families where the wife works more than forty hours a week, there is early evidence that the husband's health suffers." The sociologist adds: "Mothers who work full-time have higher levels of stress than those who do not work.[59]

I have no regrets. Seeing my son and daughter interact with others and their growth and development gives me joy.

In this day and age, there is little respect for stay at home mothers. They are considered worthless to society because they think it takes two to provide financially for a family. In order to survive, the family has been pressured by the world to think that one income is inadequate for a man to take care of his household. I do not hear many

---

[59] Ebony, p. 136-138

people speaking out about mothers staying at home to raise their children. This is not the norm in today's culture! It is mostly unheard of in the twenty-first Century. Because of the rules of this generation, you must be strong in the Lord and the power of His might in order to stand against the voices that tell you: "you cannot achieve this in the family". You may be persecuted and frowned on because you chose to take a stand against what is considered the norm by our society. Many people feel you should put your infant in daycare. There are some very good daycares. I am not against daycares, because some people do not have a choice. The ones who have a choice to stay at home or not, can consider all of the dangers, traumas, and dramas that are attached to your child being in someone else's care.

There should be joy caring for your husband and children and making sure they are healthy and stress free. Stay at home mothers are not stupid slaves, or do not have degrees, neither goals nor dreams. We do it all. We can be called accountants, doctors, lawyers, engineers, nurses, administrators, secretaries, etc. There are so many things we do daily that can demonstrate those skills. We cannot go to school to learn motherhood. You must live the life of motherhood in order to learn what is necessary to be a mother!

Being conscious of what Jesus Christ says determines "What is good, what is evil or "What is foolish", in this world. By Gods standards, being a stay at home mother is a God given responsibility.

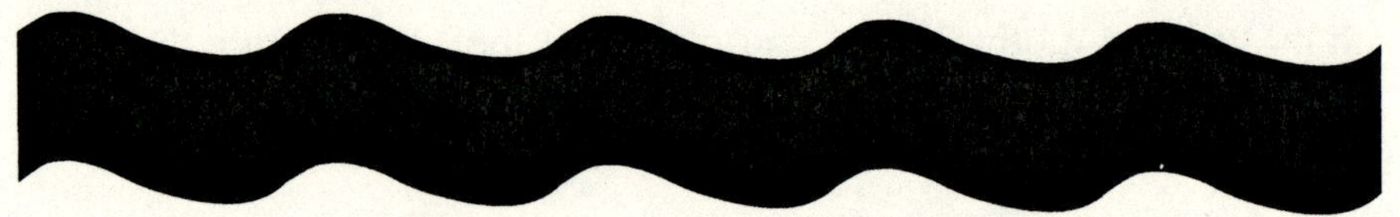

CHAPTER TWELVE

THE CHALLENGES

Sometimes there are challenges a mother may experience while breastfeeding. For an example, if your baby bites you while you are breastfeeding as my son and daughter have done; I tapped their mouth firmly once to let them know that they could not do this anymore. According to author Pamela Smith in the book Healthy Expectations, there are times when motherhood seems to be nothing but feeding the mouth that bites you![60]

This is called chastisement. Chastising my children seems to hurt me more them it does them. The Scripture instructs us to discipline our child. Just in case you do not agree, here is the Word on the matter!

---

[60] Healthy Expectations, p. 214

(Proverbs 19:18 KJV) says:

Chasten thy son while there is hope, and let thy soul spare for his crying.

By doing this, my son and daughter never bit me again, unless I was trying to force feed them when I was engorged and tried to release the milk. A word to the wise, only feed your baby when your baby is hungry, not when you are engorged with milk and hurting. You can relieve your engorged breast by placing a warm face cloth on them to soothe the pain you have. There is also an old fashion remedy where you may use warm cabbage leaves that will accomplish the same relief. You also have the option of pumping the milk from your breast.

We are often challenged with the question: “Why not give your baby cereal or other foods along with breastfeeding”? Some may say, “Babies do not get full on just breast milk”. And “They are not getting all of their nutrients to survive”. According to a number of pediatricians, some babies need cereal and baby food after six months. If you are eating properly, taking your supplements, and feeding your baby when the baby is hungry, your baby will get enough and will not need anything else.

Many people undermine breastfeeding. As I have stated previously throughout this book, please pray and read about this subject before taking anyone's advice. Educate yourself thoroughly for your own conscious sake. You will be confident with your decision to breastfeed your precious gift from God.

Most importantly, the father should be brought into understanding the benefits of breastfeeding. For this to be done successfully, he has to work along with the mother to give her support. If you do not have support from the father, you can become frustrated and loose heart for the opportunity of a lifetime, to share a closeness that only a nursing mother can have.

What about the foods you can or cannot eat while breastfeeding? I was told not to eat nuts, cabbage, citrus foods and milk products, etc., or foods that caused an allergic reaction to some babies. Yes, you do have to watch what you eat. This is a challenge that you have to determine; if you are eating healthy and mindful of the types of foods which are suggested not to be eaten, then there should not be any problems with your baby breaking out with a skin rash or any other type of reaction.

There were specific foods that I had to refrain from while breastfeeding. Yours may be different. When I ate oranges or citrus fruits, the back of my son legs would have a terrible itchy rash. In addition to that, his feet would break out in red blister type bumps. He would wake up my husband and I in the middle of the night because the blisters were itching and burning. After I figured out which foods were causing the skin problems, I stopped eating them.

You will never make the wrong decision if you consult the Lord for your infant and about your eating habits.

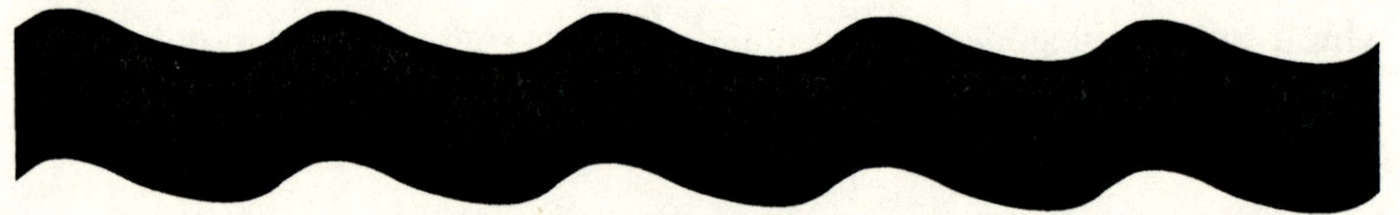

CHAPTER THIRTEEN

THE APPEAL

As a mother I realize that I have been nurtured throughout my relationship with Christ. The strength, desire, courage; the nurturing that I received came from God alone. It is amazing how God does that by his love, patience, and understanding. The nurturing comes through a relationship with Jesus Christ. Once you have a relationship with him, your thoughts will be established and your life can be stable and secure. For the understanding of something so divine; allow God, the nurturing One, to give it to you.

Here is how that can be done according to the Holy Bible, the Book of **John Chapter 3 verse 16 reads,** "For God so loved the world that he gave his only begotten son, that whosoever believes in him should not perish but have everlasting life". God does not want you condemned. He wants to have your heart and he wants to be the conductor of your thoughts.

Your response can be: Lord, I believe in your love for me. Because you love me, I want to show my love to you. Take charge of my heart. Establish my thoughts. Lord, I need you to nurture me and through Jesus your Son I make that possible. Amen!

APPENDIX

Books and Resources

The following were both referenced and footnoted in *A Champion Mother* or else sources of additional information on topics I have touched upon. While I have found something of extreme value in each of these articles, books, websites, etc., their inclusion is not necessarily an endorsement of them in their entirety.

Armstrong, Eddie, BSN., *Guide for the Breastfeeding Mother* (Columbus, OH: Ross Products Division, Abbott Laboratories, 1996).

Baumslag, Naomi, and Dia L. Michels, *Milk, Money, and Madness: The Culture and Politics of Breastfeeding* (Westport, CT: Bergin and Garvey, 1995).

Birch, William G., M.D. L.L.D. (Hon.), *A Doctor Discusses Pregnancy* (Chicago, IL: Budlong Press Co., 1995).

Clark, Adam, *The Holy Bible, containing the old and New Testament, The Text carefully printed from the most correct of the present authorized translation, including the marginal readings and parallel texts, with commentary and critical notes designed as a help to a better understanding of the Sacred Writings.* (Volume 1, the Old Testament, Genesis to Deuteronomy. New York, Nashville, Abingdon-Cokesbury Press, no date)

Eisenberg, Arlene, Murkoff, Heidi E., and Hathaway, Sandee E. B.S.N.

What to Expect When You're Expecting (New York, NY: Workman Publishing Co., Inc., 1996).

Ezzo, Gary, Buckham, Robert, *On Becoming Baby Wise* (Multnomah Publishers, Sisters, Oregon, 1998).

Fairview Health System, Wellness Center Lamaze and Breastfeeding Classes, Rocky River, OH: 1999.

Farb, JoAnn, *Compassionate Souls: Raising the Next Generation to Change the World* (New York: Lantern, 2000).

Hanson, Llars A, *Breastfeeding Stimulates the Infant Immune System*, Science & Medicine, vol.4, No. 6, Nov/Dec 1997

Huggins, Kathleen, and Linda Ziedrich, *The Nursing Mother's Guide to Weaning* (Boston: Harvard Common, 1994).

Kamen, Betty and Si, *Total Nutrition during Pregnancy: how to be sure you and your baby are eating the right stuff* (Keats Publishing Inc., 1981).

Kitzinger, Shelia, *Breastfeeding Your Baby* (New York: Knopf, 1989).

La Leche League International, *The Womanly Art of Breastfeeding* (New York: Plume, 1997)

Maire, Messenger, *The Breastfeeding Book* (New York: Van Nostrand Reinhold Co., 1982)

Mohrbacher, Nancy & Stockkk, Julie, *The Breastfeeding Answer Book* (Illinios: Schaumburg, 1997)

Promotion of Mother's Milk, Inc, *101 Reason To Breastfeed Your Child by Leslie Burby,*

(ProMom); www.promom.org; 1998-2001.

Rodriguez, Linda, M.D., *Children's Health: Problems & Solutions* (Texas, Dallas: Bruce Miller Enterprises Inc., 1996).

Sears, William, M.D., and Martha Sears, *The Baby Book: Everything You Need to* Know *about Your Baby from Birth to Age Two* (Boston: Little Brown, 1993).

Smith, Pamela, *Healthy Expectations: Preparing A Healthy Body for A Healthy Baby* (Lake Mary, Fl: Creation House, 1998).

Tanner, Lindsey, *"Moms Urged to Nurse for a Full Year"* (Chicago-Associated Press: 1997).

Tenney, Merrill, *The Zondervan Pictorial Bible Dictionary* (Grand Rapids, MI: Zondervan Publishing House, 1967).

The Plain Dealer Newspaper, *Breast feeding Cuts Risk of Cancer, Study Shows (*Cleveland, OH: Associated Press, 2001).

Worthington-Robert, Bonnie, Ph.D. and Taylor, Lynda E., M.S., *A Doctor Discusses Nutrition During Pregnancy & Breast Feeding* (Chicago, IL: Budlong Press Co., 1994).

Your Baby First Year: A Guide to Infant Growth and Development, The Enfamil Family of Formulas Guide. Evansville, IL: Mead Johnson & Co., 1998.

Zodhiates, Spiros, *The Hebrew-Greek Key Study Bible King James Version* (Chattanooga, TN: AMG Publishers, 1991).

Zondra, Hughes, *Ebony*, A Johnson Publication, *Joys of Being A Stay-At-Home Mom*,

May 2001, vol LV1, No. 7, pg. 136

Onlines Resources:

www.aboverubies.org. Breastfeeding God's Way (Article: The Power of Motherhood)

www.bestfed.com. Breastfeeding, attachment parenting, and more links to many other related subjects.

www.breastfeeding.co.uk. Jane's Breastfeeding Resources: Breastfeeding Articles, p.1, 2.

www.cdc.gov. Human Milk Banks, breastfeeding resources

www.greensboro.com. Great Women: Recognizing their leadership in American Society, past and present (News & Record's Newspaper in Education Online, 1998)

www.indiana.edu. Poison Ivy; Indiana University Health Center (Bloomington, Indiana)

www.lalecheleague.org. La Leche League. This is an excellent site with lots of wonderful information and support, plus links to other sites.

www.promom.org. 101 Reasons to Breastfeed Your Child

www.Shaklee.com. Shaklee Corporation

www.texas-midwife.com. Breastfeeding & The Bible by Larry G. Overton